Perinatal Mental Health: The Edinburgh Postnatal Depression Scale (EPDS) Manual

Second edition

John Cox, Jeni Holden and Carol Henshaw

RCPsych Publications

To Karin

© The Royal College of Psychiatrists 2014

RCPsych Publications is an imprint of the Royal College of Psychiatrists,
21 Prescot Street, London E1 8BB
http://www.rcpsych.ac.uk

British Library Cataloguing-in-Publication Data.
A catalogue record for this book is available from the British Library.
ISBN 978 1 909726 13 0

Distributed in North America by Publishers Storage and Shipping Company.

The views presented in this book do not necessarily reflect those of the Royal College of Psychiatrists, and the publishers are not responsible for any error of omission or fact.

The Royal College of Psychiatrists is a charity registered in England and Wales (228636) and in Scotland (SC038369).

Printed by Bell & Bain Limited, Glasgow, UK.

Contents

WITHDRAWN

The authors

John Cox is Professor Emeritus of Psychiatry at Keele University, UK, and was a senior lecturer in Edinburgh, and a lecturer at Makerere University in Uganda 1972–1974. He is a semi-retired consultant psychiatrist with a special interest in perinatal and transcultural psychiatry, and has published widely in these fields. He was President of the Royal College of Psychiatrists (1999–2002) and Secretary General of the World Psychiatric Association (2002–2008). He is a Founder Member and Past President of the Marcé Society. John lives with Karin in Cheltenham, close to two of their three daughters and two grandchildren. He continues to write and maintain his interests in medicine, ethics, music and hill walking.

Jeni Holden is a retired psychology lecturer and former health visitor. With John Cox and Ruth Sagovsky she developed the Edinburgh Postnatal Depression Scale. Following the research she extensively trained health professionals in the UK in the care of perinatal women. Jeni now lives in Edinburgh near one of her sons and two grandchildren.

Carol Henshaw is a consultant in perinatal mental health at Liverpool Women's Hospital and Honorary Senior Lecturer at the University of Liverpool. She was a senior lecturer in psychiatry at Keele University for 11 years and has held an Honorary Visiting Fellowship at Staffordshire University since 2003. She was awarded a Winston Churchill Memorial Trust Fellowship in 2004 and is Past President of the Marcé Society (2004–2006). She has published widely on perinatal and women's mental health.

Acknowledgements

The Edinburgh Postnatal Depression Scale is used in many countries and we wish, therefore, to thank all those international friends who have contributed so much to its development. In particular, our thanks to Ruth Sagovsky, who co-authored the first publication. Thanks also to the health visitors, doctors and midwives who helped with the research and made many useful suggestions, and special thanks to the mothers and their partners who gave us permission to quote from their interviews recorded during the counselling study.

We are grateful also to our former colleagues, in particular to Sandra Elliott and Janice Gerrard, who developed with us the evidence base for using the scale in the community and who provided so many helpful comments over the years. We wish to acknowledge the very helpful comments from Cheryll Adams, whose familiarity with the current role of health visitors in the new National Health Service structures in England has been invaluable. Finally, special thanks to Richard Bambridge, who worked with us on the project in Edinburgh and gave us his continuing support until his untimely death.

Abbreviations

BDI	Beck Depression Inventory
CBT	cognitive–behavioural therapy
CES-D	Center for Epidemiologic Studies Depression Scale
CIS	Clinical Interview Schedule
CIS-R	revised Clinical Interview Schedule
CPHVA	Community Practitioners' and Health Visitors' Association
DALYS	disability adjusted life years
DAS	Dyadic Adjustment Scale
EPDS	Edinburgh Postnatal Depression Scale
GHQ	General Health Questionnaire
GP	general practitioner
HADS	Hospital Anxiety and Depression Scale
HADS-A	Hospital Anxiety and Depression Scale, anxiety subscale
HRSD	Hamilton Rating Scale for Depression
K10	10-item Kessler Psychological Distress Scale
MADRS	Montgomery–Åsberg Depression Rating Scale
MAQ	Maternal Attitudes Questionnaire
MAMA	Meet-A-Mum Association
MSSS	Maternity Social Support Scale
NBAS	Neonatal Behavioral Assessment Scale
NCCMH	National Collaborating Centre for Mental Health
NHS	National Health Service
NICE	National Institute for Health and Care Excellence
PANDA	Post and Antenatal Depression Association
PDSS	Postpartum Depression Screening Scale
PDSS-SF	Postpartum Depression Screening Scale, short form
PHQ-9	9-item Patient Health Questionnaire
POMS	Profile of Mood States
RDC	Research Diagnostic Criteria
SAD	State of Anxiety and Depression scale
SCL-90-R	revised 90-item Symptom Checklist
SIGN	Scottish Intercollegiate Guidelines Network

SPI   Standardised Psychiatric Interview
SRQ   Self-Reporting Questionnaire
VAS   visual analogue scales
WLFLQ   Work Leisure and Family Life Questionnaire
Zung SDS   Zung Self-Rating Depression Scale

List of figures

Foreword

The Edinburgh Postnatal Depression Scale (EPDS) has become something of a 'national treasure' for perinatal mental health practitioners and researchers. Since it was first developed and described in the *British Journal of Psychiatry* in 1987, it has been used internationally in many diverse settings, cited more than 3500 times and contributed to our contemporary understanding of the fundamental importance of perinatal mental health for mothers and their families.

This manual is not only what it says on the tin. It is indeed a practical manual with helpful tips on how to use the EPDS in practice and a useful resource of translated versions of the EPDS. But it also offers a research update on depression in pregnancy and the postnatal period by wise, experienced clinicians who have used their humanist, woman-centred approach to integrate insights from other researchers and practitioners, and provides space for women's voices, with frequent use of quotes from qualitative studies to provide context and meaning to the concepts discussed.

The authors make it clear that the EPDS should not be used by health professionals as a tick-box exercise, and emphasise that health professionals who use the EPDS need to be trained in the nature, detection and treatment of perinatal depression, in understanding the experiences of women and in developing listening skills so that they can elicit and respond to psychological issues, including how to respond if women disclose suicidal ideation. There are also reminders to service managers as well as to clinicians, that health professionals including midwives and health visitors will need support to do this work.

The evidence base on interventions for perinatal depression is also provided here, including details of innovative methods such as internet-based therapy. Moreover, the authors highlight how the term 'postnatal depression' or 'perinatal depression' can be misused, sometimes with tragic consequences, such as when puerperal psychosis is mislabelled as postnatal depression, with a consequent failure of professionals to identify the high risk of psychosis in the postnatal period. Professionals caring for women in the perinatal period always need to take a proper mental health history, and the authors make clear that the EPDS is a complement to the history rather than a substitute.

This volume therefore provides an abundance of treasures inside, and will ensure that the EPDS is used wisely and thoughtfully for the benefit of women across the globe.

Professor Louise Howard
Institute of Psychiatry, King's College London

Preface to the first edition

John Cox and Jeni Holden

The Edinburgh Postnatal Depression Scale (EPDS) is a 10-item self-report scale devised as a screening questionnaire to improve the detection of postnatal depression in the community. This book is written to provide readers in different countries with updated and accessible information on the scale and its use in primary and secondary care. Appendix 1 includes the original scale and a score sheet, and Appendix 2 shows most of the foreign-language versions we are aware of.

Depressive disorders are one of the most common causes of disability worldwide. According to the 1999 World Health Report (World Health Organization, 1999), unipolar major depression accounts for 4.2% of the world's total burden of disease as measured by 'disability adjusted life years' (DALYS) and is the fifth leading cause of disability.

Postnatal depression, which affects women at a time of maximum vulnerability and can last if untreated for many years, is one of the main contributors to this disconcerting statistic. Yet, as we show in this text, the possibility of secondary prevention through early identification is consistent with the evidence base and is being actively considered by national governments in many countries, led by primary care professionals.

The EPDS was developed in the 1980s because clinical experience in both rich and poor countries showed that unipolar depression, and postnatal depression in particular, is a common disorder that causes much unnecessary misery for women and their families. We were also becoming aware that such depression can adversely affect the development and nutrition of the infant, the continuity of the marriage and the economy of the household.

Since then, worldwide communications have become almost instantaneous, women's health issues have developed a higher profile and the knowledge base of perinatal mental health and perinatal psychiatry has increased substantially. The Marcé Society (an interdisciplinary society that stimulates research and provides a forum for disseminating information about perinatal mental health) has flourished and become more truly international, and the voices of women are now more clearly heard, as qualitative research methods complement a quantitative approach and as voluntary patient and carer groups are influencing governments and so changing mental health priorities.

Within this context the EPDS has provided a timely stimulus to considering the prevention of postnatal depression. In the UK, primary care professionals are now more skilled in detecting such depression and providing a range of evidence-based therapies. The EPDS has also facilitated much epidemiological research by its use as a first-stage screening measure. Furthermore, because of its sensitivity to change over time, it can be used as an outcome measure in treatment studies.

Although the scale was devised to meet the needs of quantitative research as well as for clinical use, it has opened up an important qualitative debate about the meaning of symptoms, the equivalence of metaphor (e.g. 'things have been getting on top of me') and the cross-cultural validity of a scale developed from within a specific social context.

It is remarkable that the UK debate about the use and misuse of the EPDS should have moved on from a local consideration to a matter for a National Screening Committee, which has rightly pointed out deficiencies in the evidence base that must be addressed before national universal screening can be put firmly in place.

The response of the Community Practitioners' and Health Visitors' Association (CPHVA) has been equally committed. Health visitors, only too familiar with the consequences of untreated perinatal mental disorder, have already taken the lead role in screening for this common and treatable disorder. They have become familiar with the skills and consequences of conducting clinical assessment interviews and, in particular, recognise the usefulness of the EPDS when administered by a fully trained health professional. The EPDS does not screen for those at risk of becoming depressed in the future, but it will identify a mild depression, which can rapidly develop into a severe, prolonged disorder.

The evidence base for the optimum use of the EPDS must continue to be explored. We hope that its wider use will facilitate long-overdue treatment trials. Above all we hope that the EPDS will continue to encourage practitioners to listen to women, to take what they say and how they say it seriously, and also to collect data that will lead to a higher priority being given to perinatal mental health and women's health issues in general.

The training of obstetricians, general practitioners, midwives, health visitors, psychiatrists and psychologists is still deficient in many aspects of psychosomatic obstetrics and perinatal care. We hope that this handbook will help to change things, increasing the chances for new mothers to establish a good relationship with their infants and an optimal environment in which the children may develop.

We hope that our book will encourage researchers and clinicians across the world to develop perinatal mental health strategies and to search for ways of preventing a condition that can reduce the quality of life for the parents – and for the next generation.

Perinatal mental health is contingent on the support of society and is difficult to maintain in the presence of mental disorder. We have seen too many families break up as a result of a mental disorder at this time for the priority of these services to be overlooked, even when resources are very limited.

The EPDS was developed from experience of clinical work in health visiting and psychiatry in the UK and East Africa. It will be for clinicians to decide how and in what way this brief self-report scale, with its simple method of scoring, will continue to be used in the treatment and secondary prevention of postnatal depression.

Preface to the second edition

John Cox, Jeni Holden and Carol Henshaw

The Edinburgh Postnatal Depression Scale (EPDS) has continued to be used throughout the world by clinicians and researchers since the first edition of this book was published in 2003. Its ten items and simple scoring method have remained unchanged for almost three decades and when used as we intended the EPDS has outlasted most of its initial criticisms.

The suggestion of a second edition of our book has therefore been warmly welcomed; it has given us the opportunity to welcome Carol Henshaw as a third author. Carol was a former academic colleague at Keele University and presently works as a consultant perinatal psychiatrist in Liverpool. As a Past President of the Marcé Society she is also well placed to ensure the book's relevance to the postmodern world in which we live, and to help us make sure that the different clinical contexts in which the EPDS is used are fully recognised.

By 2030, depression is predicted to be the leading cause of disability, with only HIV/AIDS and perinatal disorders higher for low- and middle-income countries (Mathers & Looncar, 2006). In the UK there have been striking changes in the delivery of perinatal services, with an emphasis on quality standards and agreed care pathways. It is a key advance that the National Health Service (NHS) in England has included perinatal services within the remit of a separate Specialised Services Commissioning Board which was established in April 2013. In low-income countries, perinatal mental health and the impact of perinatal mental disorder on the developing infant and on educational attainment is now a more widely acknowledged public health priority.

We have updated all the chapters and their references, included a list of the 57 languages and the EPDS translations known to us, modernised the screening sections and re-emphasised the continuity of depression before and after birth in at least a third of mothers, but have left largely unaltered the balance of the book and the preface to the first edition which drew attention to humanistic values and to the need to ensure the questionnaire's cultural validity.

The book's original title has been modified to *Perinatal Mental Health: The Edinburgh Postnatal Depression Scale (EPDS) Manual* to complement our original publication in the *British Journal of Psychiatry* (Cox *et al*, 1987), which is so widely quoted.

We hope, and might expect, that new EPDS users would carefully read this updated manual before using the EPDS in their clinical work or research.

We continue to welcome correspondence and much appreciate receiving information from around the world about the scale's use, and occasional misuse. The early detection and clinical management of perinatal mental disorder, and its impact on the whole family, remains a current international priority. We expect that the EPDS will continue to be of use in facilitating this important work.

CHAPTER 1

Postnatal depression: an overview

'My husband wants another baby. The idea is quite nice, but it really frightens me to think that after having the baby I would be like this again. I wouldn't mind the morning sickness or the actual birth. It is the postnatal depression that really frightens me. I don't think I could face that again. It was horrific.' (Holden, 1988)

Introduction

Postnatal depression affects not only the quality of a woman's own life and her experience of mothering but also her infant, her other children, her partner and everyone around her, including those involved in her care. On an individual level, the experience can be devastating. Pitt (1968) noted that many of the women in his early study felt quite changed from their normal self, and most 'had never been depressed like this before'. Without help or treatment, the consequences may be long term and expensive for the women, for their families and in the demands made on healthcare resources. In severe depression, especially with psychotic symptoms, there is a risk of suicide and infanticide. *The Confidential Enquiries into Maternal Deaths in the United Kingdom* (Oates, 2001), which covered the triennium 1996–1999, first reported psychiatric causes as the leading cause of maternal deaths in the UK and this has remained the case in subsequent reports.

The term 'postnatal depression' is commonly used to describe a sustained depressive disorder in women following childbirth, characterised by:

- a low, sad mood
- lack of interest
- anxiety
- sleep difficulties
- reduced self-esteem
- somatic symptoms such as poor appetite and weight loss
- difficulty coping with day-to-day tasks.

The term was used by Vivienne Welburn (1980) as the title of her book and by Ann Oakley (1980) to describe a sustained depressive disorder occurring in women in the first year after childbirth. It was also used in the Edinburgh study (Cox *et al*, 1982) to describe women experiencing depression within 3 months of childbirth. Cox *et al* offered the conservative estimate of 13% for the prevalence of depression at that time and report that half of these women were not identified by the local primary care service. In the USA, the term 'postpartum depression' is more commonly used to describe mothers with a non-psychotic mood disorder.

Participants at a workshop in Sweden (organised by Birgitta Wickberg, Philip Hwang and John Cox) concluded that the term postnatal depression is useful to describe any depressive disorder without psychotic features present within the first year following childbirth; the limitation of the 4-week onset specifier in DSM-IV (American Psychiatric Association, 1994) and 6 weeks in ICD-10 (World Health Organization, 1992) was recognised. DSM-5 published in May 2013 (American Psychiatric Association, 2013) has extended the onset-specifier period to 6 months, but ICD-11 is not due for publication until 2015.

In the late 1970s and throughout the 1980s postnatal depression was largely considered to be a Western phenomenon, with infrequent documentation in the cross-cultural literature. This suggested that it might be a 'culture-bound' phenomenon. Possible contributing factors were thought to be the lack of social structuring of the event of childbirth, combined with a lack of accompanying ritual and support for the mother (Stern & Kruckman, 1983; Cox, 1996). Research has increasingly revealed that depression is a negative outcome of childbirth for women in diverse countries and cultures (Halbreich & Karkun, 2006).

The public health importance of postnatal depression is now more widely acknowledged in mental health policy guidance both in the UK and in other countries than formerly because of the suffering and disability of the woman and the disruption of the family at a time of maximum vulnerability. The evidence of depression having an adverse effect on the mother–infant relationship and on child development is also more widely recognised.

It is well established that postnatal depression affects at least 10% of women within the first postpartum year and that even higher rates occur in urban areas of deprivation. Cooper *et al* (1999), for example, found that a third of women in an African township in Cape Town had a serious major depressive disorder. Similarly, Cryan *et al* (2001) found that 28.6% of 944 women in a socially deprived urban area in Dublin, Ireland, had depression postnatally. The frequency of depression is much lower in cohesive island communities such as Malta (Felice *et al*, 2004) and in affluent societies with generous maternity benefits such as Sweden (Wickberg & Hwang, 1997). It is also less common in cultures with more clearly defined parental roles such as Japan (Tamaki *et al*, 1997) and Malaysia, where the majority of women still retain traditional postnatal beliefs and practices (Kit *et al*, 1997) and in countries where childbirth gives high status to the married mother (Cox, 1983).

Postnatal depression is not, however, a specific discrete disorder fundamentally different from depression occurring at other times, and our use of the term does not indicate that such depression always develops after delivery or is necessarily caused by the specific stress of childbirth. Pitt (1968) considered depression after childbirth to be 'atypical', although we ourselves did not find the symptoms different from depression at other times, for example in mothers with older children (Cox *et al*, 1996). Nor was there evidence in a Stoke-on-Trent study (Murray *et al*, 1995) that the range of depressive symptoms distinguished between early-onset (i.e. within the first 6 weeks) and later-onset depression. However, one case-record study reported that women with postnatal depression had more anxiety features and took longer to recover than women with major depression unrelated to childbearing (Hendrick *et al*, 2000).

A study by Henshaw *et al* (2004) – and subsequently by others (Adewuya, 2006; Watanabe *et al*, 2008; Reck *et al* 2009) – has confirmed, however, that severe 'postnatal blues' (see pp. 4–5) is a powerful predictor of subsequent depression: 40% of women with severe postnatal blues subsequently developed a depressive disorder. These findings suggest that the birth event can be an important neuroendocrine trigger for a more sustained depressive disorder, an idea supported by the work of Bloch *et al* (2000). They administered a gonadotrpohin-releasing hormone agonist, which suppresses the hypothalamic–pituitary–ovarian axis, to women who did and did not have histories of postnatal depression. They then gave the women supraphysiological doses of oestradiol and progesterone, mimicking the hormonal state of late pregnancy. The hormones were then withdrawn under double-blind conditions and women with histories of postnatal depression were more likely to develop mood symptoms in the withdrawal period. Cooper & Murray (1995) studied two groups of primiparous women for 5 years and found that women for whom the index postnatal episode was a recurrence of depression were at increased risk of further non-postpartum episodes but not of postpartum episodes. Women for whom the index postnatal episode was the first experience of depression were at greater risk for further episodes of postnatal depression but not for non-postpartum episodes. They concluded that their findings supported the use of postnatal depression as a specific diagnostic entity.

In about 15% of cases, postnatal depression has an antenatal onset and depression in pregnancy is as common as it is postpartum. Gavin *et al* (2005) reported that incidence of new-onset depression in pregnancy (14.5%) was the same as the incidence in the first 3 months postpartum, and Bennett *et al* (2004) observed prevalence rates of 7.4%, 12.8% and 12.0% for the first, second and third trimesters respectively. Depression during pregnancy is associated with a number of adverse fetal outcomes including increased activity, delayed growth, preterm birth and low birth weight (Field *et al*, 2006).

There have to date been several Cochrane reviews published on the treatment of antenatal depression and the prevention of postnatal depression. The review of psychosocial and psychological interventions for the treatment of antenatal depression concluded that as the only trial (of interpersonal psychotherapy) reviewed was so small, the authors could not make any recommendations (Dennis *et al*, 2007). The review of non-biological treatments found insufficient evidence of their efficacy to support the use of massage therapy or acupuncture (Dennis & Allen, 2008).

Progestogens do not prevent postnatal depression and are associated with depressive symptoms in some women. Progesterone has not been formally tested in a randomised trial (Dennis *et al*, 2008). Nortriptyline showed no benefit over placebo, and although sertraline did seem to prevent a recurrence or extend the time to recurrence in some women who had previously had a postpartum depressive episode, the numbers in the trial were very small (Howard *et al*, 2005). Dennis & Creedy (2004) reviewed 15 trials of psychological or psychosocial interventions for the prevention of postnatal depression, concluding that there was no benefit over usual care. A Health Technology Assessment systematic review of psychological and psychosocial interventions for the prevention of postnatal depression which will update this is currently underway and due to report in 2014.

Other postnatal psychiatric disorders

Postnatal depression is generally distinguished from puerperal psychosis by its later onset following childbirth (4–6 weeks) and by the absence of florid delusions, hallucinations and gross behavioural disturbance that can characterise puerperal psychosis. Research findings suggest that puerperal psychoses are linked in their aetiology and prognosis to bipolar mood disorders (Chaudron & Pies, 2003). The risk of recurrence of puerperal psychosis following subsequent pregnancies and bipolar disorder after childbirth is at between 1 in 2 or 1 in 3 (Kendell *et al*, 1981a; Wieck *et al*, 1991). Although rare (2 per 1000 deliveries), puerperal psychoses can have devastating consequences for the mother (suicide) (Oates, 2003) and the infant (infanticide) (Oates, 2003; Spinelli, 2003). Their optimal management usually requires the full resources of a perinatal mental health team with access to a purpose-built mother and baby unit, as recommended by the Joint Commissioning Panel for Mental Health (2012) in England and Wales, Scottish Intercollegiate Guidelines Network (SIGN) in Scotland (Scottish Intercollegiate Guidelines Network, 2012) and in other national guidelines. With comprehensive treatment, however, the prognosis is usually good, although there is a high risk of recurrence. Women affected should therefore be closely monitored in all subsequent pregnancies and after delivery, when appropriate prevention strategies should be in place and a clear management plan provided by specialist perinatal mental health teams, communicated to all involved in their care.

Postnatal blues describes the transitory mood disturbances (emotional lability and crying) found in at least two-thirds of women in the first week postpartum and particularly on day 5 (Cox *et al*, 1982; Henshaw, 2003). An understanding of postnatal blues is important for a number of reasons, including the following:

1   They are distressing and perplexing for the mother and her family, and there is therefore a need for an explanation of their causes and for support and reassurance.
2   Severe blues can be difficult to distinguish from the premonitory signs of puerperal psychosis and from the early onset of non-psychotic postnatal depression.
3   Increased understanding of the neuroendocrine causes of postnatal blues will contribute to knowledge about the effect of gender steroids on central neurotransmitter systems and provide a window for further understanding of postnatal mood disorder.

The relationship between postnatal disorders is shown in Fig. 1.1, which illustrates the maintaining factors ('vicious circles') of postnatal depression and how the lack of culturally sanctioned family support can both cause and be a consequence of a prolonged depressive disorder at this time.

Other important psychiatric disorders found in the puerperium include anxiety disorders: panic disorder, obsessive–compulsive disorder, post-traumatic stress disorder and generalised anxiety disorder. The EPDS is sensitive to anxiety (Matthey *et al*, 2013*a*), as is the subscale EPDS-3A (Swalm *et al*, 2010). However, there have been no comparison studies with standard anxiety measures. The EPDS may not detect the less common disorders such as schizophrenia, alcoholism, substance misuse or an organic confusional state. However, some of the depressive episodes indentified by the EPDS may be bipolar depression (Wisner *et al*, 2013).

Women's narratives

Mothers themselves often describe their depression and its effects graphically. In tape-recorded interviews conducted after a randomised

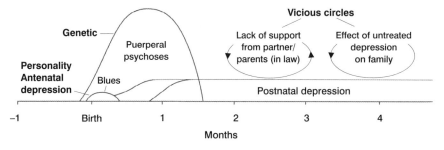

Fig. 1.1   Causal and maintaining factors of postnatal depression (after Cox, 1998).

controlled trial of counselling by health visitors (Holden, 1988), women expressed their feelings in the following way:

> 'I have never felt like that in my life before. Nobody could speak to me because I would burst into tears at the least thing. I took an extreme dislike to everybody in this world except my baby. I wanted everybody to go away, I was interested in nothing.'

> 'It was terrible. It was like someone else taking over. I wasn't the same person any more. I didn't recognise myself. It wasn't me, that was what I kept saying. It wasn't me.'

> 'It was absolutely ghastly. It felt as if there was a physical weight inside that was dragging me down. I was pulling it around all the time; everything was an effort.'

Another mother told us that something had 'got a hold of her' which she knew was serious and required medical help. In an earlier study, in at least a half of the women who developed depression, the disorder lasted for a year and sometimes merged into a second postnatal depression that followed a subsequent pregnancy (Cox *et al*, 1984). Many women clearly recalled postnatal depression several years later.

Effects on interactions with infants

Postnatal depression occurs when heavy demands are placed on women's resources and when infant learning and development are taking place.

> 'Mothers of young infants, especially when it is their first child, must adjust to their baby and learn to understand the infant's communications and needs. This task is more difficult if the mothers are feeling despondent, fatigued and overwhelmed by the responsibilities attendant upon transition to parenthood... [T]he sadness, irritability and social withdrawal that characterise depressed women compromise their ability to provide a sensitive, nurturing environment for their babies.' (Campbell & Cohn, 1997: p. 166)

After completing our counselling intervention study, many woman told us of the effect that depression had had on their relationship with their infant. One woman had seriously feared harming her baby, and constantly fantasised while bathing him about how easy it would be to push his head under the water. Others said:

> 'It was lonely and I felt as if I was inside this box, just all by myself, with nobody to talk to and nobody to help me. I started taking my anger out on [my baby]. I never hit him, but I grabbed him. Or I used to ignore him, let him scream, shut him away. I wasn't loving him like a mother should.'

> 'It really bothered me to be depressed when I had such a lovely baby, it didn't seem fair to her. I never stopped loving her, but I couldn't express it. I was withdrawn into myself. I liked the baby but I wasn't interested in her. I just did things automatically and I wouldn't remember doing them. It was as if I wasn't really there. I felt I was a failure as a mother.' (Holden, 1988)

One health visitor became concerned that another mother showed little interest in her baby, leaving him entirely to her sister to look after. This woman told me that she had felt she was not a good enough mother, and that the baby would know this and reject her.

The accounts cited earlier were retrospective (between 9 and 12 months postpartum), describing how the women had felt in the early months. In a controlled study, Jennings and colleagues (1999) found that more than half of mothers with depression had a fear of being alone with their infant and felt an inability to care for the infant. Indeed, 41% of mothers with depression compared with 7% of control mothers admitted to thoughts of harming their infant. A later study reported universal intrusive thoughts of the infant coming to accidental harm and almost half of the sample of mothers with depression experienced intrusive thoughts of harming their infants. This was predicted by high parenting stress and low social support, and there was no association between these thoughts and aggressive parenting (Fairbrother & Woody, 2008).

Adverse effects on the mother–infant relationship and the feelings of both mother and baby are well documented. Murray et al (1996) found, in a comparison with well women, that at 2 months postpartum, mothers with depression were less sensitively attuned to their infants and were less affirming and more negating of infant experience. Murray et al suggested that persistent patterns of withdrawn behaviour may in this way be set up in the baby which could limit subsequent experience and development, even after the mother has recovered and is responding more affectionately.

Research groups have looked at the ways in which these mother–infant interactions are disturbed. A preliminary study by Kaplan et al (1999) of the long-term impact of postnatal depression on mother–child interaction demonstrated for the first time that 4-month-old babies react with far less interest to the speech of mothers with depression. The tape-recorded voices of mothers without depression were more likely to stimulate their infants' interest and the time they spent focusing on an abstract pattern. Edhborg et al (2001) suggested that the young children of women with high EPDS scores develop 'representations' of their mother and of their interactions with her as being less joyful than do the children of mothers without depression, and that these representations may remain beyond the period of the mother's depressed mood. Depressive symptoms in both mothers and fathers is negatively associated with positive enrichment activity with the child such as reading, singing songs and telling stories (Paulson et al, 2006).

Persistence of effects on children of mothers with depression

There is considerable evidence of a sustained adverse affect of maternal depression on the infant's later cognitive development and behaviour (reviewed by Grace et al 2003). Disturbances in early mother–infant interactions were found to be predictive of poorer infant cognitive outcome at 18 months of age (Cooper & Murray, 1997). In children 3.5 years of age and at school entry both postnatal and more recent maternal depression were associated with significantly raised levels of child disturbance, particularly among boys and those from lower social class families (Sharp *et al*, 1995; Sinclair & Murray, 1998). These unwanted effects may persist even longer and may be mediated by chronic or recurrent maternal depression. In a study of long-term sequelae in the children of mothers who had depression at 3 months postpartum, for example, Hay *et al* (2001) found that 11-year-old children, especially boys, had significantly lower IQ scores, more attentional and reading problems, greater difficulties in mathematical reasoning and were more likely to have special educational needs than children of mothers who had not had postpartum depression. Although several studies have found boys to be particularly vulnerable, chronic maternal depression persisting into the second postnatal year in one study was associated with lower psychomotor and cognitive development, but this study found no infant gender differences (Cornish *et al*, 2005). There is some evidence, however, that such effects can be changed by an intervention to help the mother during depression (Murray *et al*, 2003; Poobalan *et al*, 2007).

Postnatal depression has also been associated with poor infant growth in both high- and low-income countries (reviewed by Stewart, 2007), but a more recent large multicentre study in Europe found no relationship between infant growth measurements and maternal postnatal depression in high-income countries (Grote *et al*, 2010). Field's review noted that postnatal depression is associated with compromised feeding practices (especially breastfeeding), sleep routines, attendance at well-child visits, immunisation rates and safety practices (Field, 2010).

Fathers and postnatal depression

In the past most research into perinatal distress has concentrated on the mother: surprisingly little attention has been paid to fathers around the time of childbirth.

Postnatal depression in the mother commonly has a profound effect on her partner and on their relationship. Fathers may themselves develop depression. In Birmingham, UK, Ballard *et al* (1994) studied 200 couples postpartum and found that the prevalence of depression (ascertained by the earlier 13-item EPDS) in fathers was 9.0% at 6 weeks after the birth and 5.4% at 6 months. As expected, mothers had a significantly higher prevalence of caseness at both 6 weeks and 6 months postpartum than fathers had, but fathers were significantly more likely to be cases if their partners had depression. In a longitudinal study in Portugal, Areias *et al* (1996*a*) found that in the first 3 months postpartum, nearly a quarter of the women shown to be at risk in pregnancy developed depression, in contrast with less than 5% of their partners. In the next 9 months, however, men were more prone to developing depression than previously and their depression tended to follow the earlier onset of depression in their partner. Condon (2006) has reviewed the psychological adjustment of expectant fathers, their response to a partner with a mental health problem and the impact of the relationship with the partner and the father's mental health on father–infant interaction.

Matthey *et al* (2001), who validated the EPDS for use with fathers, found a relatively low level of depression in men compared with the level in their postnatal partners and this has been confirmed by other studies (e.g. Escribà-Agüir & Artazcos, 2011). However, distress was more likely in the father when the mother was also distressed, and depression in fathers is associated with an increased risk of disharmony in the partner relationship even when maternal depression is controlled for (Ramchandani *et al*, 2011). New fathers' depression rates have been found to be twice the rate in healthy controls in Denmark (Madsen, 2006) and in the USA (Paulson *et al*, 2006). One meta-analysis notes substantial heterogeneity among rates in the 43 studies included and reports a meta-estimate of 10% (Paulson & Bazemore, 2010).

Fathers scoring above threshold on the EPDS in the antenatal and postnatal period in the Avon Longitudinal Study of Parents and Children were more likely to have children with psychopathology, and those fathers with depressive symptoms postpartum only had sons with higher rates of conduct problems (Ramchandani *et al*, 2008).

The important role of fathers in supporting their partners through pregnancy and beyond is increasingly recognised. According to Holopainen (2002), the father's functioning is central, as new mothers with depression receive more support from their partner than from any other individual, including medical staff. Field (1998) found that fathers' support may also shield the infants of mothers with chronic depression from negative outcomes. Edhborg *et al*'s small observational study in 2003 showed that in families where mothers had persistent depressive mood, their infants had established joyful relationships with their fathers, and infant–father attachments were secure.

The mother's relationship with her partner may, of course, contribute to rather than ameliorate her low mood. In a review in 2006, Fisher *et al* identified factors related to maternal depression, including a poor relationship with the father, his being unavailable at the time of the baby's birth and his provision of what is perceived by the mother to be insufficient emotional or practical support including low participation in infant care. Other risk factors identified include the father holding rigid gender-role expectations or being controlling or violent. Imaginative interventions may help the couple to understand and perhaps change unhelpful behaviours.

After our counselling study, fathers were asked about their experiences during their partners' depression:

> 'It was terrible. No matter what you do you are wrong. She was awfully quick tempered; things she would normally laugh about just make her mad.'

'She had changed a lot. Before, if we had a lovers' tiff, in the finish we would start laughing at how stupid we were. But now, the least little thing and she starts to cry. I've been kicked out of the house hundreds of times, but I never went.'

'I could see there was something wrong with her, and she was telling me it was the depression, but I used to say to myself "Is this just an excuse she is using, is she really tired of me, does she really want me to go?"' (Holden, 1988)

Although in this study we had not set out to look at depression in fathers, several of the partners of women in the study themselves spoke of feeling depressed, and it was clear that the wife's depression caused considerable disruption to the relationship of the majority of couples. In tape-recorded interviews, both men and women spoke of a loss of affectionate closeness:

'If he puts his arms around me I absolutely shudder. I say "Oh, Dave don't come near me!" And it is pretty frightening because I have never been that way. All the time that I've known Dave we used to sit and cuddle each other, we were always very close, but now he sits over there and I sit over here.' (Holden, 1988)

Many couples who had been in the group that received counselling reported that this support had sustained or even improved their relationship. Without help, however, depression can lead to relationship breakdown. In the control group, one husband left his wife completely because he could not cope with the unpredictability of her moods. Another left for 3 months but came back after his wife had recovered from her depression. Almost a year after his first baby was born, another husband said that he had often thought of leaving:

'It was great before the baby came. But now...I'd be as well being a monk. What matters in a marriage, well, it's nine-tenths of a marriage, is sex and, well...and love. And if you can't get even a cuddle, nobody's going to stay around.' (Holden, 1988)

Couples told us that they were totally unprepared for the possibility of depression and claimed that it had not been explained or even mentioned in antenatal preparation classes. It is hoped that the increasing awareness of health professionals will improve both prenatal and postnatal information given to new parents.

Clinical perspectives

The presentation of postnatal depression was usefully summarised by Brice Pitt (1968) in his pioneer study of London women. He emphasised the way in which depressive symptoms were often coloured by the mother's relationship with her baby and the need to understand additional stressors caused by mothering. Pitt described postnatal depression as follows:

'[The women experience] tearfulness, despondency, feelings of inadequacy and inability to cope – particularly with the baby...Guilt was mainly confined to self-reproach over not loving or caring enough for the baby...Many felt quite changed from their usual selves, and most had never been depressed like this before.

Depression was almost invariably accompanied, and sometimes over-shadowed, by...anxiety over the baby [which] was not justified by the babies' health...

Unusual irritability was common, sometimes adding to feelings of guilt. A few patients complained of impaired concentration and memory. Undue fatigue and ready exhaustion were frequent, so that mothers could barely deal with their babies, let alone look after the rest of the family and cope with housework and shopping.

Anorexia...was present with remarkable consistence. Sleep disturbance, over and above that inevitable with a new baby, was reported by a third of the patients.' (Pitt, 1968)

Identifying postnatal depression

This manual describes how the EPDS can improve the detection of postnatal depression in the community, sometimes as an additional component of a clinical interview. In an earlier publication (Cox, 1989) it was suggested that one or all of the following could alert the obstetrician, midwife, health visitor or general practitioner (GP) that a mother has possible clinical depression:

- a complaint of feeling low, worried, fatigued or having severe sleep difficulties
- constant complaints of somatic symptoms such as headaches, abdominal pain or breast tenderness, without an adequate physical cause
- an expressed fear that the doctor or health visitor will be excessively critical of her mothering ability, and may even be considering taking away her baby
- excessive concern about the baby's health and preoccupation with minimal feeding difficulties
- continuous over-solicitousness and immediate response to the baby's demands
- unexpected failure to attend a postnatal clinic or child health clinic
- a baby who is failing to thrive and crying excessively.

O'Hara (1995) has described the clinical presentation in the USA in the following way:

'About day 3 postpartum, Mrs Jones's mood began to sink. She said that her low mood felt almost like physical pain. She also reported feeling anxious and irritable at this time. During the period of her depression, which lasted at least 2 months, she completely lost her appetite. She woke up during the night and could not get back to sleep. She commented that it was almost like not falling asleep. She had no energy and lost interest in most things. Mrs Jones reported feeling guilty; in particular, she believed that she wasn't a good mother, and she blamed herself for her son's colic. She also had extreme difficulty in

11

concentrating. Finally, she found that her work and family relationships were "impaired by her depression". Despite both her mother and husband urging her to seek help for her depression, she did not. At 6 months postpartum, she was still reporting a moderate level of depressive symptomatology.' (p. 9)

Confirmation of the diagnosis

If a mother is assessed by a health worker as being 'possibly depressed' or if she has a high score on the EPDS, then specific enquiry should be made about the presence or absence of the following depressive symptoms or complaints:

- *Depressed mood* Most women recognise when they are down, sad, depressed, low-spirited or 'blue'. Asking the question 'How do you feel in your spirits these days?' will usually elicit this crucial information. The health professional can then determine the extent to which this depressed mood is a break from the usual mood state, and establish how long the mood has lasted and how distressed the mother is. A depressed mood that has lasted for at least 4 weeks and is accompanied by other symptoms of depression would strongly suggest that the mother has clinical depression.
- *Excessive anxiety* Although being anxious (fearful, worried) can occur in the absence of depressed mood, if anxiety is present it should be regarded as coexisting with depression unless shown not to be so. It is wise to assume that any mother who is anxious is also likely to have depression.
- *Lack of interest and pleasure in doing things* Anhedonia is a hallmark of depression. The lack of interest may show itself through an unusual disinterest in usual activities or social interaction or in resuming sexual relations – libido is often non-existent.
- *Early morning wakening* Early morning wakening when not caused by a noisy baby or a restless partner is characteristic of depression; when consistently present and prolonged it is especially typical of the depressed phase of bipolar disorder. Initial insomnia, when the mother is kept awake by rounds of worrying thoughts or by an exaggerated need to listen to any sound from her baby, may be another sign of a depressive illness.
- *Ideas of not coping, self-blame and guilt.*

The clinical skills required to determine the presence or absence of these symptoms of depression can usually be acquired during supervised undergraduate or postgraduate training or from a post-qualifying refresher course for primary care health professionals.

Women with depression who have fixed delusional ideas of guilt or self-blame congruent with their depressed mood are best described as having severe depression. It is very important to identify this group of women in primary care because they may have an increased risk of self-harm and may require treatment with antidepressants and immediate referral to a specialist team.

The ICD-10 primary care criteria for a depressive disorder (F32) (World Health Organization, 1992) can be recommended for use by GPs. These criteria specifically identify women who have given birth as being at high risk.

Causes

The possible causes of postnatal depression can usually be ascertained only after a full clinical history has been obtained from the mother and her family. A biopsychosocial approach should be used when establishing causes, and this includes understanding the way that the social environment may influence the expression of genes and the likelihood of adverse life events. The causal domains involved are illustrated in Fig. 1.2.

Present preoccupations of society with postnatal depression and the popularity of the label may reflect a greater concern about women's health issues in general, the status of childbearing in society and the increased vulnerability of modern families. In almost all societies depression can be identified postpartum, but the meaning of this condition for the mother and her family will vary. Local popular explanations may include biological (hormonal), social (lack of support) and psychological factors (e.g. 'my baby is making me depressed') (Fig. 1.3).

In low- and middle-income countries or in societies riven by warfare, a mother's inability to obtain basic essentials (food, clothes and warmth) for herself or her children may provoke additional hardship, exclusion, hopelessness and eventually clinical depression.

There is no simple, single cause for postnatal depression.

Robertson *et al* (2004) reviewed the literature and calculated effect sizes:

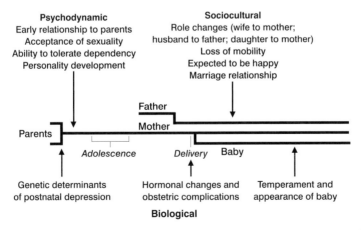

Fig. 1.2   Possible causal factors in postnatal depression (after Cox, 1986: p. 39).

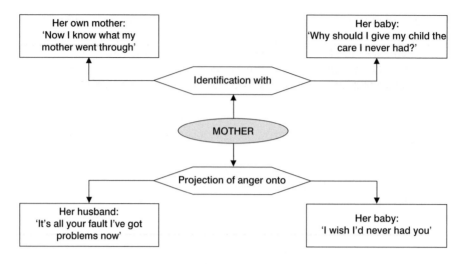

Fig. 1.3 Identification and projection: common psychological defence mechanisms in the puerperium (after Cox, 1986: p. 35).

- strong/moderate risk factors:
  - depression or anxiety during pregnancy
  - life events
  - social support
  - history of depression
- moderate risk factors:
  - neuroticism
  - marital relationship
- small risk factors:
  - socioeconomic status
  - obstetric factors.

Findings from our own studies suggest that the following are associated with postnatal depression in mothers: the previous personality of the mother (always being a 'worrier'); a history of mental disorder; earlier loss of the mother's own mother; severe postnatal blues; giving up work reluctantly; and a poor relationship with the mother's mother (see also Holden, 1991).

There is now greater understanding of the way that oestrogen receptors influence central neurotransmitter systems. Genetic studies (Coyle *et al*, 2000) have found an increase in the 12 allele of the serotonin (5-HT) transporter gene in women with a susceptibility to bipolar disorder who develop puerperal psychosis. More recent work has shown linkage with chromosomes 16p13 and 8q24 (Jones *et al*, 2007).

Future studies of brain function might show the way in which a crying baby, fractious husband or intrusive mother-in-law could modify brain functions in the postpartum period, and how these difficulties in a susceptible mother might provoke mental disorder. The evidence for such a specific neurobiological trigger for postpartum mood disorder is at present circumstantial, but the finding (Henshaw *et al*, 2004) that women with severe blues have a 1 in 4 risk of developing subsequent major depression is a strong pointer to pursuing this line of research enquiry.

However, the results of the International Transcultural Study of Postnatal Depression show that when women themselves are asked to describe the cause of unhappiness before and after childbirth, they give explanations almost entirely in the social domain (Oates *et al*, 2004). Indeed, it is popularly assumed that the primary cause of postnatal mood disorder is the meaning that women attach to events and to the lack of instrumental and psychological support. Interestingly, today only rarely do women attribute postnatal mood disturbances to a disorder of brain function caused by hormonal changes.

Gender of the infant may be an important factor to consider in some cultures (e.g. Chandran *et al* 2002; Abiodun, 2006).

It is nevertheless possible that physiological changes in the mother in the immediate postpartum months do increase the likelihood of emotional disturbances, but that the emotions experienced are contingent on the memories laid down in earlier formative relationships, on the nature and availability of social support and, in particular, on the meaning for the mother of giving birth to a dependent infant.

Caring for women with postnatal depression

The main use of the EPDS in routine clinical work is to assist in the secondary prevention of postnatal depression by identifying the disorder as early as possible so that therapy can be initiated. Supportive counselling by a primary care worker such as a health visitor, midwife or practice nurse can be particularly effective for women with mild depression (Holden *et al*, 1989; Morrell *et al*, 2009; see also other studies reported in Chapter 5). Assistance from a mental health worker with a special interest in perinatal mental disorder is necessary for women who continue to have depression despite counselling, for those at risk of suicide and in situations in which the baby is at risk of neglect or physical abuse by the mother. Women who have developed depressive disorder with psychotic features (delusions of guilt, self-blame or persecution) will also need care from a specialist perinatal team. If other members of the family also have mental health problems or the stress has affected older children, then the skills of a family-oriented psychiatric team are very important. In this context, the use of the care programme approach and the development of a care plan to coordinate multiprofessional working that includes the mother and her family are useful. For women with severe mental disorder or those recovering from psychosis, multiprofessional management strategies, including child protection and the identification of a keyworker, are recommended.

The present book does not describe in detail the treatment options for women with severe postnatal depression who require specialist help from secondary services. Other sources (e.g. National Institute for Health and Clinical Excellence, 2007; Henshaw *et al*, 2009; Scottish Intercollegiate Guidelines Network, 2012) must therefore be consulted for this information. The principles of the treatment approach, however, do not differ substantially from the treatment of depression at other times, although the social context of new parenting, the presence of a dependent infant and the specific features of a risk assessment in the puerperium need always to be considered.

In Chapter 5 we give particular emphasis to the benefit of counselling by primary care workers. It is important to stress, however, that this approach alone is likely to benefit only women with mild to moderate depression and that the combination of counselling with antidepressant medication is necessary for women with severe depression as recommended by the National Institute for Health and Care Excellence (NICE) (National Institute for Health and Clinical Excellence, 2009).

CHAPTER 2

The origins and development of the Edinburgh Postnatal Depression Scale

Origins of the EPDS

In the early 1980s, the limitations of existing self-report questionnaires for use in community samples were beginning to be recognised. Philip Snaith (1983), for example, had acknowledged the need to modify existing scales for use in specialist settings; and Channi Kumar (1982), in *Motherhood and Mental Illness*, recognised there was a need for

> '...some form of simple self-administered scale...for use in antenatal and postnatal settings, to pick out potential cases of women with depression and anxiety. Existing questionnaires contain questions which are dissonant with the woman's pregnant or parturient state and, on the other hand, questions about her mental state, which take account of her condition, are lacking.' (p. 112)

In Edinburgh at that time the serious limitations of existing self-report scales had become very apparent to us. Although we used the best available scale in our prospective study (Cox, 1983) – the Anxiety and Depression Questionnaire (SAD) of Bedford & Foulds (1978) – and although it had the advantage of brevity and few somatic items, it failed to detect any increase in these symptoms in the first postpartum weeks, and the recommended cut-off score was completely inappropriate for use during pregnancy (Cox, 1983). Of the 13 pregnant women with a score of 6+, only 3 had any form of mental disorder, and some items lacked face validity for childbearing women. We concluded:

> 'If these difficulties with the SAD are replicated by others using different self-report questionnaires, then the implications for the reliable detection of neuroses in childbearing women are considerable. It might for example be necessary to re-design or re-validate self-report scales specifically for use during pregnancy and again for use in the puerperium.' (p. 6)

The intent of the grant application to the Scottish Home and Health Department in 1983 was therefore to develop and validate a screening scale specifically for use with childbearing women in the community, and also to carry out an intervention study by health visitors. In the proposal the limitations of existing scales was emphasised, as well as the published evidence that perinatal depression, and postpartum depression in particular, caused distress to the mother, was a threat to family cohesion and had an adverse effect on the growing infant. The relevance to the proposed research of Pitt (1968) and Kumar & Robson (1978) as well as our prospective prevalence study in Edinburgh was emphasised. Pitt's finding that of 305 women attending routine obstetric clinics in East London, 33 (10.5%) developed a depressive illness 6 weeks after childbirth, and 4% remained depressed for at least 12 months, was seminal to the project. Likewise, Kumar & Robson's (1978) Camberwell study: they had interviewed 100 married women with the Standardised Psychiatric Interview (SPI) and found that 19 had psychiatric morbidity in the puerperium, which in 13 women had an onset after childbirth. Similarly in Scotland, of the 103 women included in a more representative antenatal sample, 13 women were found to have sustained postpartum depression, and a further 17 women, shorter depressive episodes (Cox *et al*, 1982). We also used the SPI, which was familiar from John Cox's earlier Ugandan research. Each mother was interviewed twice before delivery, and at 1 week and 4 months after childbirth. The clinical characteristics of the 13 women with sustained postnatal depression were found to be very similar to those described by Pitt; and we particularly noted that in 9 women the onset had followed childbirth. The mothers commonly reported self-blame, inability to cope with family responsibilities, sad mood and were often tearful and anxious.

Thus existing self-report scales for depression such as the SAD (Bedford & Foulds, 1978), the Beck Depression Inventory (BDI) (Beck *et al*, 1961) and the General Health Questionnaire (GHQ) (Goldberg, 1972) all had serious limitations for use with pregnant and postpartum women. Women might endorse (tick) the somatic items on the scales because of the physiological changes of childbearing (e.g. weight gain, breathlessness, tachycardia), and childbearing women can disclose normal worries. Sleep difficulty as a symptom of depression is difficult to evaluate when sleep is being disturbed by the baby.

In 1983 it was noted that such 'false positives' in self-report questionnaires might reduce the reliable detection of neurosis in pregnant and postpartum women, and that scales specifically for use during pregnancy and in the puerperium might be needed (Cox, 1983). Zigmond & Snaith (1983), who developed the Hospital Anxiety and Depression Scale (HADS), also recognised the need to modify existing self-report scales for use in specific clinical situations. Williams *et al* (1980) emphasised that questionnaires validated for use on hospital samples should be revalidated when used in the community.

Thus, by the mid-1980s the need to develop a depression scale specifically validated for use by childbearing women was apparent and increasingly compelling.

Validating the EPDS

At the outset of our project it was recognised that a questionnaire for use with childbearing women would need to be simple to complete and acceptable to people who did not regard themselves as unwell. Furthermore, the healthcare worker administering the scale may not have any specialised training in psychiatric disorders. Finally, the new scale would need to have satisfactory validity and reliability, and be sensitive to changes in the severity of depression over time.

Clinical experience when assessing and treating women with postnatal depression was used to identify possible items from questionnaires such as the SAD, HADS and BDI. Items that lacked face validity (i.e. that would not have been understood by childbearing women or might have been inappropriate at this time, e.g. 'I can enjoy a good book or radio or television' or 'I feel as if I am slowed down') and somatic items (misleading as indicators of depression) were discarded. We then selected 30 items – which included several of our own construction – to pilot with women, who were asked to comment about the wording and the order of the items.

We eventually agreed on 13 items that we thought likely to detect mothers with clinical depression. The resultant questionnaire was then validated (Cox, 1986) on a sample of 60 postnatal women, who completed the 13-item scale and were interviewed by the psychiatrist Ruth Sagovsky using the Clinical Interview Schedule (CIS) (Goldberg *et al*, 1970). The diagnosis of depression using major and minor Research Diagnostic Criteria (RDC) (Spitzer *et al*, 1978) was then established. The 13-item scale was found to distinguish satisfactorily between women with and without depression. A factor analysis, however, showed not only a 'depression' factor that explained 46% of the variance but also another factor that loaded on three items ('I have enjoyed being a mother' and the two irritability items). We therefore realised that the 13-item scale could be shortened to 10 without impairing its effectiveness. This shortened 10-item scale (named the Edinburgh Postnatal Depression Scale) had no specific item about mothering the baby or about irritability, a development that later widened the potential use of the scale to other populations.

A second validation of the 10-item version was carried out on a sample of 84 postnatal women who were taking part in an ongoing study of health visitor counselling (Fig. 2.1) (Cox *et al*, 1987). The shortened scale identified all women with definite major depression and two of every three women with probable major depression at a cut-off of 12/13. Of the 11 women with definite minor depression, only 4 had a false-negative score. Although this cut-off resulted in 11 false positives, 6 of these women had several depressive symptoms without fulfilling all RDC for clinical depression. Interestingly, three women with a psychiatric diagnosis other than depression all scored below the cut-off.

19

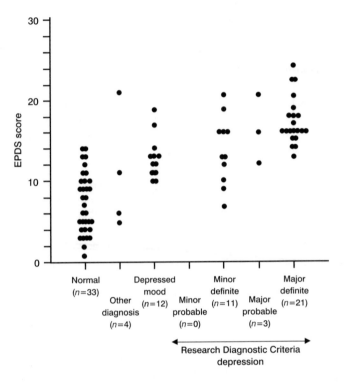

Fig. 2.1 Validation of the 10-item Edinburgh Postnatal Depression Scale (EPDS; Cox *et al*, 1987).

The sensitivity of the EPDS (the proportion of women with RDC depression who were true positives) was 86%, and the specificity (proportion of women without RDC depression who were true negatives) was 78%. The positive predictive value (the proportion of women above the threshold on the EPDS ($n = 41$) who met RDC for depression ($n = 30$)) was 73%. These findings suggested that the rate for failing to detect women with depression could be reduced to under 10% by using a lower cut-off of 9/10. This was the cut-off that we recommended in our initial publication of the EPDS for use as a first-stage screening measure. Gibson *et al* (2009) from the Oxford National Perinatal Epidemiology Unit have, however, correctly pointed out in their schematic review the heterogeneity of many recent validation studies of the EPDS and the need for more research on its psychometric properties in the community, and especially in naturalistic settings. We endorse this sentiment particularly with regard to its validity during pregnancy. We are also aware that there is a need for more definitive controlled prevalence studies of perinatal depression which will provide a more firm base for the development of comprehensive community perinatal services. Interestingly, Gibson and colleagues, on the basis of their analysis, endorse the recommended cut-off scores we suggested in our original Edinburgh validation study and as first published in 1986 (Cox, 1986).

Reliability

The split-half reliability of the 10-item EPDS was 0.88 and the standardised coefficient 0.87. (The split-half reliability was obtained by dividing items on the scale into half, and the halves were then compared; a high correlation suggested that the items were measuring the same characteristics.) The sensitivity to change in severity of depression over time was established by comparing EPDS scores obtained at two interviews separated by a 3-month interval. This showed that the EPDS can be used to detect changes in the level of depression over time, so widening its use as an outcome measure in intervention studies.

The three women with a false-negative score each had other family members present when they were interviewed. We recommend that the EPDS is optimally completed when other family members are not present, as women may exaggerate or minimise their problems in these circumstances. The 10-item EPDS was found to be very acceptable to most of the women and, as important, to their health visitors. Another advantage of the scale was its brevity and simplicity of scoring.

These findings, together with our clinical experience, suggested that the EPDS would be useful in detecting postnatal depression in the community as well as in research projects. A cut-off of 9/10 was likely to detect almost all cases of depression, with very few false negatives. This cut-off score is particularly useful in a research project in which the EPDS is the only measure used or when it is used as a first-stage screening scale to identify possible depression. Another advantage of the EPDS in epidemiological studies is that it can elicit a high response rate (95–97%) when sent by post, especially if there had been previous contact with the research team and there is follow-up of women who do not initially respond (Murray & Carothers, 1990; Roy *et al*, 1993).

In the community, the EPDS is useful in the secondary prevention of postnatal depression by identifying the early onset of depressive symptoms. It can be administered by a trained health visitor, practice nurse or midwife at a postnatal or child health clinic or on a home visit. When using the EPDS in primary care settings as a component of a screening programme, the 9/10 cut-off may be over-inclusive, so a cut-off of 12/13 is often recommended. It should be remembered that the EPDS screens only for depression and that women who score below the cut-off may, none the less, have clinical depression.

The scale is best administered by a health professional who is familiar with mental health problems and has had training in their evidence base. A woman with a high score or an unexpectedly low score should be further assessed by a health professional and/or referred to a GP, mental health nurse, psychologist or psychiatrist. A mother with profound depression might not grasp the meaning of the items; others may wish to cover up their disability or fear stigma or the shame of not coping.

Readability

The EPDS has been assessed as at or below US 6th grade (equivalent to age 11 or 12), which is recommended for public documents (Logsdon & Hutti, 2006).

Comparisons with other scales

Several studies have compared the performance of the EPDS with other depression questionnaires for use in the postnatal period and during pregnancy.

Given the findings of some of the studies cited, it is likely that the differences in performance may reflect differences in the population investigated.

We developed the EPDS because other depression measures available at that time were problematic for use with postnatal women living in the community. Other scales may be developed in the future, perhaps specific to a local population, particularly if the population is from a diverse cultural background. However, we recommend the continued use of the EPDS because it is widely used in different countries and therefore allows useful comparison between findings – and it is now the most frequently validated method to identify women with postnatal depression (Hewitt et al, 2009).

Beck Depression Inventory

In the UK (Wales), Harris et al (1989) compared the EPDS and the BDI in their abilities to identify women who had major depression according to DSM-III criteria (American Psychiatric Association, 1980). The sensitivity of the EPDS was 95% and its specificity 93%. They concluded that the performance of the BDI was markedly inferior in this application, with a sensitivity of 68% and specificity of 88%.

In a Canadian study, Lussier et al (1996) found a low concordance between the BDI and the EPDS. Their analysis revealed distinct response patterns belonging to divergent subgroups, suggesting that the two instruments were differently attuned to the various aspects of the presentation of postnatal depression.

More recently, Lam et al (2009) compared the two scales in pregnant women in Peru, concluding that both showed good internal consistency and an acceptable Pearson correlation. Su et al (2007) found that the optimal cut-off for the EPDS in pregnant Taiwanese women was 13/14 for the second trimester and 12/13 for the third trimester. There was no variation by trimester for the BDI.

The scales' performance has also been studied in Chinese men with postnatal depression (Lai *et al*, 2010). The sensitivity and specificity were 91% and 97% respectively for the EPDS (with a 10/11 cut-off) and 100% and 81% respectively for the BDI.

In a study of low-income African American postpartum women, Tandon *et al* (2012) concluded that the EPDS and BDI-II performed equally well and that the optimum cut-off for the EPDS was 10/11. It also performs as well as the BDI when administered via the internet (Spek *et al*, 2008).

Hospital Anxiety and Depression Scale

Another Welsh study (Thompson *et al*, 1998) found that the EPDS was superior to the HADS in identifying RDC-defined depression and similar to the observer-rated Hamilton Rating Scale for Depression (HRSD) (Hamilton, 1960), which it also matched for sensitivity to change in mood over time.

An Australian group (Condon & Corkindale, 1997) found little agreement between the EPDS, the depression subscale of the HADS, the Zung Self-Rating Depression Scale (Zung SDS) (Zung, 1965) and the depression subscale of the Profile of Mood States (POMS) (McNair & Lorr, 1964). The authors concluded that this poor level of agreement might reflect the different emphasis in the item content of the questionnaires.

General Health Questionnaire and Center for Epidemiologic Studies Depression Scale

In France, Guedeney *et al* (2000) compared the EPDS with the GHQ-28 and the Center for Epidemiologic Studies Depression Scale (CES-D) (Radloff, 1977), and suggested that the EPDS was better at identifying depression in postnatal women with anhedonic and anxious symptomatology, but less satisfactory for women with psychomotor retardation. Navarro *et al* (2007) concluded that both the EPDS and GHQ were valid instruments to detect postnatal depression, anxiety and adjustment disorders in their study of women at 6 weeks postpartum, whereas Logsdon & Myers (2010) reported the EPDS to perform better in a study of adolescent mothers. When studied in women who had miscarried, Lee *et al* (1997) observed that both scales had good sensitivity and specificity, concurrent validity and internal consistency, although the EPDS only detected major depression, whereas the GHQ detected both depression and anxiety disorders.

Kessler Psychological Distress Scale

When the Kessler Psychological Distress Scale (K10) was compared with the EPDS against a DSM-IV diagnosis of depression in screening pregnant women in rural India, both scales performed equally well (Fernandes *et al*, 2011).

Zung Self-Reporting Depression Scale and Symptom Checklist-90-Revised

Although Condon & Corkindale (1997) reported little agreement between the EPDS and Zung SDS, a study of 50 Austrian postnatal women taking part in an international epidemiological study who scored 7 or more on the German version of the EPDS found that it performed equally well (Muzik *et al*, 2000). The authors compared the EPDS, the German Zung SDS (with a clinical cut-off score of 50) and the depression and anxiety subscales of the revised 90-item Symptom Checklist (SCL-90-R) (Derogatis & Cleary, 1977) with a cut-off *T*-score of 63. Diagnoses of depression and anxiety were made using the Structured Clinical Interview for DSM-III-R. The authors reported that the German version of the EPDS screened reliably for postnatal depression but that further research was needed to create screening measures for postpartum anxiety disorders.

Self-Reporting Questionnaire

A study in rural Ethiopia reported that the EPDS performed less well than the Self-Reporting Questionnaire (SRQ) (Hanlon *et al*, 2008), but a later study in Addis Ababa observed that in an urban setting the EPDS performed better (Tesfaye *et al*, 2010). Pollock *et al* (2006) observed a better performance by the SRQ in a literate urban population in Mongolia. When the EPDS was compared with the SRQ in non-literate and impoverished women in Pakistan, both instruments were effective but the health workers administering them preferred to use the SRQ because of its simpler format (Rahman *et al*, 2005). Both instruments were equally valid when used in a Brazilian sample at 3 months postpartum (Santos *et al*, 2007a).

Patient Health Questionnaire

The 9-item Patient Health Questionnaire (PHQ-9) is commonly used in UK primary care. Flynn *et al* (2011) found few differences in the scales' performance when assessing major depression in pregnant and postpartum women in a US psychiatric out-patient setting. However, another study found some concordance between the scales when used to screen postpartum women, though 17% of scores were discordant. This was predicted by being younger than 30 and having a lower educational level (Yawn *et al*, 2009). Hanusa *et al* (2008) found the EPDS and the short form of the Postpartum Depression Screening Scale (PDSS-SF) more accurate than the PHQ-9. The EPDS and PHQ-9 were used with a cut-off of 9/10 and the PDSS-SF with a cut-off of 13/14. A community-based study of postpartum women (most of whom were not literate) in Ghana reported that although internal consistency was equivalent across the scales, the PHQ-9 had better test–retest reliability and criterion validity when compared with the EPDS (Weobong *et al*, 2009).

Postpartum Depression Screening Scale

In the USA, Cheryl Beck developed a screening measure, the Postpartum Depression Screening Scale (PDSS) (Beck & Gable, 2001). This scale, developed from qualitative research, was compared with the EPDS and the BDI, and validated against a DSM-IV diagnostic interview. She found that the PDSS yielded the highest combination of sensitivity (91%) and specificity (72%) of the three instruments and concluded that researchers and clinicians need to be aware of the differential sensitivity of depression instruments that are supposed to be measuring the same construct. Also in the USA, Hanusa *et al* (2008) compared the 7-item PDSS, the EPDS and PHQ-9. They concluded that the EPDS was the most accurate scale and that the EPDS and PDSS were more accurate than the PHQ-9. Chaudron *et al* (2010) screened young Black women in an urban US setting with the EPDS, BDI and PDSS. Although all three scales performed equally well as continuous measures, the optimal cut-off for detecting major depressive disorder with the EPDS was ≥9, and ≥7 for major or minor depression.

Visual analogue scales

A small study of 34 women (McCoy *et al*, 2005) compared scores on Kendell's visual analogue scales (VAS) (Kendell *et al*, 1981) at 15–21 days after delivery and the EPDS at 4 weeks postpartum. Responses on all 6 VAS items were significantly correlated with EPDS scores and regression analysis showed 61% of the variability of EPDS scores was explained by the VAS questions (McCoy *et al*, 2005).

Other uses of the EPDS

The EPDS is not specific only to detecting depression in the puerperium. It can also be used to screen for depression occurring at other times:

- pregnancy (Murray & Cox, 1990; Green & Murray, 1994; Evans *et al*, 2001; Josefsson *et al*, 2001; Jomeen & Martin, 2007; Berginka *et al*, 2011; Rubertsson *et al*, 2011)
- after miscarriage (Lee *et al*, 1997)
- terminal illness (Lloyd-Williams *et al*, 2000)
- fathers (Ballard *et al*, 1994; Areias *et al*, 1996b; Matthey *et al*, 2001; Lai *et al*, 2010; Tran *et al*, 2012). Edmondson *et al* (2010) observed that optimum sensitivity and specificity in fathers was at a cut-off score of >10, whereas in Vietnam (Tran *et al*, 2012) it was 4/5. Moran & O'Hara (2006) developed a version which can be completed by the partner of a postnatal woman to provide a perspective beyond the woman's self-report or, conversely, a maternal report of her partner's mood (Fisher *et al*, 2012).
- adoptive parents (Gair, 1999)

- peri-menopausal women (Becht *et al*, 2001)
- non-postnatal women (Cox *et al*, 1996)
- mothers and fathers of toddlers (Thorpe, 1993)
- mothers with intellectual disability (Gaskin & James, 2006).

The scale can be administered by computer with adequate acceptability and performance (Glaze & Cox, 1991; Spek *et al*, 2008).

We re-emphasise that the EPDS is not a measure of general psychiatric morbidity and may not detect other common perinatal disorders.

CHAPTER 3

International and cross-cultural issues

When establishing a perinatal mental health service it is always necessary to consider the local sociocultural context of childbirth and for health professionals to be culturally competent. In this way the likelihood that the EPDS is used inappropriately in different cultures and languages is diminished.

Translations

The EPDS has been translated into 57 languages and used in clinical work and research in all regions of the world. Appendix 2 contains many of these translations. This proliferation suggests that the identification of perinatal mothers with mental health problems has become a more significant public health priority.

The EPDS facilitates international and cross-cultural research as a first-stage screening questionnaire in prevalence studies and assists primary care workers to monitor the effectiveness of screening programmes and record outcomes in intervention trials. There are, however, important caveats to consider when using any translation of a questionnaire outside the culture and language in which it was developed. The EPDS, for example, is not a checklist of common depressive symptoms, and cross-cultural comparisons of EPDS scores can be misleading.

When planning to use the EPDS in a cross-cultural study therefore, it is helpful to consider both the 'etic' (when the culture is studied from an outside perspective) and the humanistic 'emic' approach, derived from an inside perspective of the local language and cultural attitudes. As suggested by Laungani (2000), different assumptions and techniques are often required to understand fully depressive disorders in unfamiliar cultures and this is of particular importance for perinatal mental disorders which are embedded in cultural customs, values and beliefs. Kumar (1994) has summarised this key point:

> 'The way in which the impact (of childbirth) is felt by the individual parent must, to some extent, be shaped by the ways in which that parent's society

and culture organises its response to parenthood, as well as by the structure of the family into which the child is born.' (p. 250)

Thus in studies of postnatal depression in Uganda and Scotland (Cox, 1999) the need to understand local 'folk' causes of depression as well as the range of available traditional treatments and the explanation for the choice of presenting symptoms was immediately apparent to the research team. For example, Ugandan women were more likely to describe somatic symptoms and less likely to express feelings of personal responsibility for the development and nurture of the baby. Furthermore, the range of postpartum support was also strikingly different for African and Scottish mothers: Ugandan mothers were often part of a large family group and a third were co-wives. Traditional naming ceremonies were common in Uganda and were an important family occasion. At the time of our study, Scottish mothers were more likely to consider biomedical causes of perinatal depression (such as changes in hormones) and to express feelings of guilt.

Flaherty and colleagues (1988) have helpfully summarised the way in which these sociocultural considerations need to be taken into account when translating a questionnaire from one language to another. They have suggested that attention should be given to the following dimensions:

1   content equivalence: the content of each item of the instrument should be relevant to the phenomena of each culture being studied
2   semantic equivalence: the meaning of each item should be the same in each culture after translation into the language and idiom, written or oral, of each culture
3   technical equivalence: the method of assessment (e.g. pencil and paper or interview) should be comparable in each culture with respect to the data that it yields
4   criterion equivalence: the interpretation of the measurement of the variable should remain the same when compared with the norm for each culture studied
5   conceptual equivalence: the instrument should measure the same theoretical construct in each culture

In the study of depression in Punjabi-speaking Sikh women in Wolverhampton, Clifford et al (1999) considered each of these five dimensions. For example, to determine semantic equivalence, each EPDS statement (and each word used) was examined to establish whether or not the meaning and idiom were the same in Punjabi as in English. For technical equivalence, the Punjabi EPDS was tape-recorded to ensure that women who needed verbal rather than written assessment would be approached in the same way.

Validation studies

In general, the EPDS has satisfactory validity when translated into most other European languages, although not all such validation studies and translations fully satisfy the five dimensions of Flaherty *et al* (1988). A list of those languages into which the EPDS has been translated (and when known the published reference to a validation study) is shown below and overleaf, and many of these complete EPDS translations are included in Appendix 2. Readers should be aware, however, that not all of these translations have been adequately validated or their reliability established.

A recent systematic mapping of evidence from low- and lower-middle-income countries, including the EPDS and other scales, noted that only 40% of the studies reported that the translation used had been validated for that population and country (Coast *et al*, 2012).

Validated translations

- Amharic (Hanlon *et al*, 2008)
- Arabic (United Arab Emirates: Ghubash *et al*, 1997; Morocco: Agoub *et al*, 2005)
- Bangla (Gausia *et al*, 2007)
- Chichewa (Stewart *et al*, 2013)
- Chinese (Hong Kong: Lee *et al*, 1998; Taiwan: Heh, 2001; Teng *et al*, 2005; mainland China: Wang *et al*, 2009; Lau *et al*, 2010)
- Dutch (Pop *et al*, 1992)
- Farsi/Persian (Montazeri *et al*, 2007; Kheirabadi *et al*, 2012)
- French (Guedeney & Fermanian, 1998; Quebec, Canada: Des Rivières-Pigeon *et al*, 2000)
- German (Austria: Herz *et al*, 1997; Bergant *et al*, 1998; Muzik *et al*, 2000)
- Greek (Thorpe *et al*, 1992; Leonardou *et al*, 2009; Vivilaki *et al*, 2009)
- Hebrew (Katzenelson *et al*, 2000)
- Hungarian (Töreki *et al*, 2013)
- Igbo (Uwakwe & Okonkwo, 2003)
- Italian (Carpiniello *et al*, 1997; Benvenuti *et al*, 1999)
- Japanese (Okano *et al*, 1996, 1998, 2005; Yoshida, *et al*, 2001)
- Konkani (Patel *et al*, 2003)
- Kurdish (Ahmed *et al*, 2012)
- Lithuanian (Bunevicius *et al*, 2009)
- Malay (Rushidi *et al*, 2002; Mahmud *et al*, 2003; Kadir *et al*, 2004)
- Maltese (Felice *et al*, 2006)
- Mongolian (Pollock *et al*, 2006)
- Nepali (Regmi *et al*, 2002)
- Norwegian (Eberhard-Gran *et al*, 2001; Berle *et al*, 2003)
- Portuguese (Portugal: Areias *et al*, 1996a; Brazil: Da-Silva *et al*, 1998; Santos *et al*, 2007b)
- Punjabi (Clifford *et al*, 1997, 1999; Werrett & Clifford, 2006)
- Samoan (Ekeroma *et al*, 2012)
- Shona (Chibanda *et al*, 2010)
- Sinhala (Rowel *et al*, 2008)

- Spanish (Chile: Jadresic *et al*, 1995; Peru: Vega-Dienstmaier *et al*, 2002; Spain: Ascaso Terrén *et al*, 2003; Garcia-Esteve *et al*, 2003; Mexico: Alvarado-Esquivel *et al*, 2006)
- Swedish (Lundh & Gyllang, 1993; Wickberg & Hwang, 1996*a*)
- Tamil (Benjamin *et al*, 2005)
- Thai (Pitanupong *et al*, 2007)
- Tongan (Ekeroma *et al*, 2012)
- Turkish (Aydin *et al*, 2004)
- Twi (Weobong *et al*, 2009)
- Vietnamese (Matthey *et al*, 1997; Tran *et al*, 2011)
- Yoruba (Adewuya *et al*, 2006)

Not validated against standardised diagnostic interview

- Afaan Oromo (source unknown)
- Czech (Dragonas *et al*, 1996)
- Dari (Shafiei *et al*, 2011)
- Estonian (source unknown)
- Filipino/Tagalog (Small *et al*, 2003)
- Finnish (source unknown)
- Hindi (Banerjee *et al*, 2000)
- Icelandic (Thome, 1992, 1996, 1999)
- Indonesian (source unknown)
- Kannada (Fernandes *et al*, 2011)
- Khmer/Cambodia (Fitzgerald *et al*, 1998)
- Korean (Kim & Buist, 2005)
- Macedonian (source unknown)
- Malagasy (Rhandawa *et al*, 2009)
- Myanmar/Burmese (source unknown)
- Polish (Bielawska-Batorowicz, 1995)
- Romanian (Wallis *et al*, 2012)
- Russian (Glasser *et al*, 1998)
- Serbian (source unknown)
- Slovenian (M. Blinc Pesek, personal communication, 2003)
- Somali (source unknown)
- Urdu (Bannerjee *et al*, 2000)
- Xhosa (de Bruin *et al*, 2004)

Explanation for lower cut-off EPDS scores in translations

Owing to these and other similar considerations, it is not surprising that validation studies using French (Guedeney & Fermanian, 1998), Chinese (Lee *et al*, 1998), Swedish (Lundh & Gyllang, 1993; Wickberg & Hwang, 1996*a*), Maltese (Felice *et al*, 2006), Italian (Carpiniello *et al*, 1997;

Benvenuti *et al*, 1999), Japanese (Okano *et al*, 1998) and Vietnamese (Tran *et al*, 2011) translations recommend a lower cut-off score for optimum sensitivity than that found in our original study. These differences may be explained by differing sample sizes or the timing of the postpartum interview and also by difficulties in translating English idioms. For example, in the UK the item 'Things have been getting on top of me' is commonly construed as 'I have felt overwhelmed by everyday tasks or events'. This has a different meaning even in North American English. Again, 'The thought of harming myself has occurred to me' is generally recognised by British women as implying suicidal thoughts, but it could be interpreted as fear of harm occurring through an accident such as falling over.

For such reasons, the use of the EPDS and its technical and conceptual equivalence in many languages is not established. For example, there were particular difficulties expressing in Punjabi items referring to anhedonia (the lack of pleasurable anticipation) and the concept of blaming oneself unnecessarily. Importantly, using the EPDS in a culture in which there is uncertainty about the nature of clinical depression and the extent to which it can be reliably assessed may be inappropriate, and could lead to premature recommendations about its effectiveness. Translations of the EPDS need to be tested in new studies to determine their usefulness in research and as a basis for providing services to women in different countries and cultures.

The scale has nevertheless been used with various diverse populations, such as Brazilian women of low income in Niteroi (Da-Silva *et al*, 1998) and in women following miscarriage in Hong Kong (Lee *et al*, 1997), and as an outcome measure in a trial of the preventive effectiveness of antenatal information in Japan (Okano *et al*, 1998). The validated Portuguese translation of the EPDS was used in Porto to investigate the comparative incidence of depression in both fathers and mothers during the woman's pregnancy and after childbirth (Areias *et al*, 1996a). It is interesting to note that multilingual health workers orally translated the EPDS to women speaking six different South African languages at a postnatal clinic in Johannesburg, where it was validated against DSM-IV (American Psychiatric Association, 1994) criteria for depression (Lawrie *et al*, 1998). In Austria, Bergant *et al* (1998) translated the scale and validated it against ICD-10 criteria for depression (World Health Organization, 1992) at 5 days postpartum in an Innsbruck hospital. Although we consider 5 days to be too soon to administer the scale, the authors reported it to be valid, reliable and 'application friendly' in this language.

The original English version of the EPDS has been validated for use in North America (O'Hara, 1994: pp. 161–162; Stuart *et al*, 1998), and it is extensively used in Australia in both research and clinical practice. It has been validated on an Australian sample by Boyce *et al* (1993). Barclay & Kent (1998) have questioned both the use of the EPDS with new immigrant mothers in Australia and the problems of conceptualising extreme misery in this population as 'depression'. They argue that a narrow approach to 'medical aetiology' may fail to include the sociocultural aspects of postnatal depression experienced by non-English-speaking immigrant women. However, Barnett *et al* (1999), discussing their studies of immigrant Vietnamese and Arabic women in New South Wales, Australia, cogently observed:

> 'Screening for postnatal depression results in more non-English-speaking women being identified and thus offered a service than if such screening does not occur. We disagree with the view that the term "postnatal depression" necessarily implies any aetiology ... Work by our unit, as well as others around the world, indicates that the psychosocial and cultural aspects related to distress in new immigrant mothers is being recognised and acted upon' (p. 203).

Conceptual models and world views

In our experience, to work effectively in perinatal mental health requires that health professionals adopt an integrative biopsychosocial- and relationship-based approach to healthcare delivery, and are aware of the shifting valances of family dynamics which may be partly hidden (Cox, 2007, 2012). In religious or secular societies having an understanding of perinatal spiritual practices and religious beliefs, which may give meaning to the birth event, can be useful in the management of some patients.

Hanlon (2008, 2012) has illustrated the relevance of these themes to establishing perinatal services in Ethiopia, where the EPDS was found to have inadequate psychometric properties in rural communities. Interestingly, Coast *et al* (2012) in their review of postnatal depression and poverty in low- and lower-middle-income countries found that 44.7% of studies were from South Asia, and of the third (38.3%) of studies from sub-Saharan Africa, more than half came from Nigeria. They observed that the majority of studies were undertaken in a relatively affluent urban setting, despite the known high rates of untreated depression in rural areas (e.g. Vietnam: Fisher *et al*, 2012) and the predicted rise in the urban poor in low- and lower-middle-income countries, where 1 in 3 urban dwellers live in slums.

The association of perinatal mental disorders with later cognitive impairment in children (Rahman *et al*, 2013) and with maternal suicide in low- and lower-middle-income countries will continue to increase awareness that the training of community health workers (including traditional birth attendants) in the recognition and management of perinatal mental disorder is a legitimate priority that will save lives and enhance the educational and economic prospects for the society.

CHAPTER 4

Using the Edinburgh Postnatal Depression Scale in clinical settings: research evidence

Does using the EPDS increase detection of perinatal depression?

Health visitors in our original counselling intervention (where health visitor–patient ratios allowed close contact with mothers whose infants were under 6 weeks) were asked to indicate whether they believed that women in their case-load were experiencing depression at their 6-week visit. The women later completed the EPDS. Despite knowing the women well, the health visitors failed to identify 60% of the women who obtained high EPDS scores at 6 weeks and were subsequently found to have depression at a psychiatric interview at about 3 months postpartum. Other UK researchers (e.g. Hearn et al, 1998), who set out specifically to determine the efficiency of the primary care team in identifying postnatal depression in women, found that using the EPDS gave an almost threefold increase in the numbers of women identified with depression.

Overseas studies have also shown that EPDS screening can increase detection rates. In Sweden, where child healthcare nurses pay regular home visits and where staff/patient ratios are considerably higher than in the UK, Wickberg & Hwang (1996b) found that health professionals identified less than half the women found to have depression, and that only a third of the mothers that were identified had spontaneously indicated their feelings. Also working in Sweden, Bågedahl-Strindlund & Monsen Borjesson (1998) found that very few women with postnatal depression were identified in routine care. In both Swedish studies, the EPDS was well accepted by both mothers and nurses, and its use significantly increased the number of identified cases.

Three studies in North America examined the ability of health professionals to detect depression with or without the EPDS. Schaper et al (1994) interviewed physicians and midwives taking part in a community study in Wisconsin to determine whether using the EPDS would increase practitioner awareness and treatment of postnatal depression. Of the professionals interviewed, 83% reported that the EPDS had increased their awareness of the condition and 92% had referred patients with high EPDS scores for treatment. At the Mayo Clinic in Minnesota, Georgiopoulos and colleagues (2001) implemented universal screening with the EPDS in all community postnatal care sites over a 1-year period. The rate of diagnosis of postnatal depression increased significantly following the introduction of EPDS screening. Evins *et al* (2000) compared the efficacy of routine clinical evaluation with that of EPDS screening in a residency training programme practice in Asheville, USA. Over 1 year, 391 patients were assigned either to screening with the EPDS or to a control group that had only spontaneous detection during routine clinical evaluation. The authors reported impressive results: the incidence of detection of postnatal depression using the EPDS was 35.4% compared with only 6.3% during routine clinical evaluation. They concluded that the EPDS is an effective adjunct to clinical interview for diagnosis of postpartum depression and that its use should be considered in residency training.

Barnett *et al* (1993) in Sydney, Australia, asked 100 mothers of infants consecutively admitted to a mothercraft residential facility to complete the EPDS. Of these 100 women, 39 scored above the cut-off point for likely major depressive disorder, only 1 of whom had been identified as having postnatal depression prior to the infant's admission.

Training health visitors to screen with the EPDS, develop a therapeutic relationship and provide a psychological intervention to women scoring below threshold at 6 weeks postpartum reduced the risk of them scoring over threshold at 6 months after delivery (Brugha *et al*, 2011).

Acceptability of the EPDS

During the 2.5 years it took to collect our data, we gained useful information about the acceptability of the EPDS. The scale was administered routinely at about 6 weeks postpartum to all women attending baby clinics in the five participating health centres. The health visitors reported that most women readily accepted screening and that with some re-adjustments to clinic procedures, administration could be absorbed into routine practice. An added reported advantage was that generalised use of the scale resulted in raised awareness among all members of the primary healthcare team, and also among the women themselves and their families, of the possibility of emotional distress or depression occurring at this time and of the importance of providing the opportunity for women to talk about their feelings. Although we have heard of instances of individual women being reluctant or even refusing to complete the scale, this has usually been for personal reasons, or because it has been insensitively presented. For example, one woman in our three-centre study felt oppressed by being asked to fill in an EPDS at the baby clinic because she had already been given one at her postnatal visit to the hospital (Gerrard *et al*, 1994). Another woman was already receiving hospital treatment for depression.

In 2003, Shakespeare *et al* found that 54% of 39 women had found EPDS screening to be 'unacceptable' and that issues of fear of stigma as well as inappropriateness of the screening venue were raised. The authors posited that results could suggest that a majority of women are distressed by the EPDS. This study was, however, small (39 women in total) and the screening was not conducted at a home visit. In our original counselling intervention, when we asked women to comment specifically about their response to the EPDS, the majority reported that it had been a relief to be asked about their feelings. Being asked to complete the questionnaire was usually taken to indicate that the health professional was concerned about their personal well-being and not only about their status as the mother of an infant (Holden, 1991). One mother said:

> 'Being told I was depressed helped in so many ways. It meant I could tell other people when they asked how I was. I was amazed how many people said they had had it themselves. Before, I couldn't tell anyone, I just pretended I was fine. I thought no one would understand. But everyone seemed to have a story about someone they had known who was depressed. If everyone was more open about it, people could help each other more.' (Holden, 1988: p. 95)

Overall, the EPDS has proved its acceptability to women in published studies conducted in a range of different geographical and sociological areas. In earlier studies in the UK, Taylor (1989) in Aberdeen, Cullinan (1991) in Hertfordshire and Angeli & Grahame (1990) in Walton-on-Thames all reported that most women had no objection to completing the scale. In Cambridge, the EPDS was posted to 702 women 6 weeks after they had given birth, and the authors concluded that a return rate of 97.3% indicated impressive evidence of the scale's acceptability to the women (Murray & Carothers, 1990). Researchers in other countries have also reported favourably on both detection rates and the acceptability of the EPDS in clinical studies (e.g. New Zealand: Webster *et al* (1994) and Holt (1995); Sweden: Lundh & Gyllang (1993) and Wickberg & Hwang (1997); Montreal, Canada: Zelkowitz & Milet (1995); Iceland: Thome (1991).

More recently, Buist and colleagues (2006) assessed the acceptability of routine screening for perinatal depression as part of a large study involving 43 hospitals across Australia. They surveyed 860 postnatal women and 916 health professionals after 3 years of routine antenatal and postnatal use of the EPDS. Overall, 90% of the women found the EPDS easy to complete, and 85% had no difficulties completing it. The researchers found that discomfort with screening was significantly related to having a higher EPDS score. A majority of health professionals reported that using the EPDS was comfortable and found it useful. The authors concluded that routine EPDS screening is acceptable to most women and health professionals. They also pointed out that sensitive explanation, along with staff training and support, is essential in implementing depression screening.

Gemmill *et al* (2006) also aimed to measure acceptability in a survey of a large community sample in Victoria, Australia, with a high representation of clinically depressed women. They used postal, telephone and face-to-face surveys with 479 respondents, some of whom had tested positive for depression. The EPDS was found to have good acceptability for both women with depression and those without. The researchers concluded that 'women's views on the desirability of postnatal depression screening appear to be largely independent of personal level of comfort with screening'.

Legitimising feelings

Some professionals believe that informing a woman that she has depression may increase the severity of depressive symptoms or that she might view the term 'postnatal depression' as stigmatising. Elliott (1994) argued cogently:

> 'Properly explained, "postnatal depression" labelling, when women are at the bottom of the spiral, may remove "depression about depression"...Labelling when at the early or subclinical depression level of the spiral may actually create "depression about depression" if the label is perceived as failure.' (p. 223)

Thome (1991) found that Icelandic mothers who scored high on the EPDS did not see their distress as 'mental disturbance', and neither did the nurses who administered the scale and supported them. The Nurses in fact admired some of their strength in living through very difficult life situations and not showing more distress than they actually did.

Two early studies in primary care showed that depression that has been recognised has a better outcome than that which is missed. Freeling (1992) found that unrecognised depression lasts longer, and Ormel *et al* (1990) showed that the beneficial effect on outcome of recognition by a GP of a mental health problem was mediated only to a small extent by treatment, and they speculated that recognition itself had beneficial effects. In a review of therapeutic interventions, Malan *et al* (1975) found that many patients with depression are helped by a single assessment interview. Such improvement may be due to the fact that the person's distress has been shared with and validated by another person (Goldberg, 1992).

One of the women who took part in our health visitor counselling intervention trial expressed cogently the relief it had been to have her depression recognised, and how this has in itself led to her subsequent ability to seek and accept help and support from others.

> 'Being told I was depressed helped in so many ways. It meant I could tell other people when they asked how I was. I was amazed how many people said they had had it themselves. Before, I couldn't tell anyone, I just pretended I was fine. I thought no one would understand. But everyone seemed to have a story about someone they had known who was depressed. If everyone was more open about it, people could help each other more' (Holden, 1988: p. 95).

Antenatal research and the EPDS

Many researchers have found that depression is common in pregnancy (e.g. Atkinson & Rickel, 1984; Watson *et al*, 1984; Ancill *et al*, 1986; Gotlib *et al*, 1989; O'Hara *et al*, 1990; Johnstone *et al*, 2001; Matthey *et al*, 2001). Green (1998), who presented EPDS scores from 1272 women, found antenatal dysphoria to be at least as prevalent as postnatal dysphoria and the majority of women had higher EPDS antenatal than postnatal scores. She also maintained that antenatal EPDS scores were fairly good predictors of postnatal scores, as did Josefsson *et al* (2001).

It is relevant to ask whether routine antenatal screening would be a useful predictor of postnatal depression, allowing scarce resources to be allocated to those at higher risk. Murray & Cox validated the EPDS for antenatal use in 1990, and it has since been used in several antenatal studies (e.g. Appleby *et al*, 1994; Green & Murray, 1994) and in the Avon Longitudinal Study of Parents and Children (Evans *et al*, 2001). Analysis of the predictive value of an antenatal EPDS is, however, controversial. In Chile, Jadresic *et al* (1992) found that women mainly had antenatal or postnatal depression, but not both. Evans *et al* (2001) also found that only a small proportion of women had depression both before and after the birth. In the UK, Watson *et al* (1984) and Brugha *et al* (1998) reported similar findings.

Should the EPDS be used as a routine screen in pregnancy?

It is clear from the research that many pregnant women do develop depression; indeed, the Avon study (Evans *et al*, 2001) found that more women had depression during pregnancy than after the birth. Detecting depression and offering treatment may be important for both the pregnant mother and her infant and for their future well-being. Research also suggests that psychopathology may have important effects on the intra-uterine environment because of increased cortisol levels (Tcixeira *et al*, 1999). It may also affect subsequent mothering behaviour: Green & Murray (1994) found that women who had scored high on the EPDS in pregnancy were less likely postnatally either to attempt or to persist with breastfeeding, more likely to view their babies as being 'more difficult' than other babies and more likely to perceive life as more difficult since the birth.

The beyondblue National Postnatal Depression Program is an impressively large prospective cohort study into perinatal mental health, conducted in all six states of Australia and the Australian Capital Territory. As part of the study, data on risk factors for postnatal depression were gathered antenatally and depressive symptoms measured postnatally between 2002 and 2005 (Milgrom *et al*, 2008). Pregnant women were screened for symptoms of depression at antenatal clinics using the EPDS and a psychosocial risk factor questionnaire that covered demographic and psychosocial information.

Antenatal depression together with a history of depression and a low level of partner support were the strongest antenatal predictors of a raised postnatal EPDS score. Antenatal depressive symptoms appeared to be as common as postnatal depressive symptoms. Previous depression, current depression/anxiety and low partner support were found to be key antenatal risk factors for postnatal depression. Limitations of the study were felt to be the use of the EPDS as the measure of depressive symptoms rather than a clinical interview, and the rate of attrition between antenatal screening and the collection of postnatal follow-up data. It could surely hardly have been otherwise with such a huge undertaking and despite these limitations much valuable data were collected. The EPDS was well accepted and the authors suggested that: 'current depression/anxiety (and to some extent social support) may be amenable to change and can therefore be targeted for intervention' (Milgrom et al, 2008).

Simply administering the EPDS in pregnancy may have positive benefits. Clark (2000) found that by focusing on the needs of the mother, not only was low emotional well-being identified, but it also provided both mothers and health professionals with an opportunity to discuss emotional health, regardless of the antenatal EPDS score. Matthey & Ross-Hamid in Sydney, Australia, were interested that a few postnatal studies have shown that many women when re-tested a few weeks later no longer score 'high' on depressive measures, and decided to explore this further with antenatal women (Matthey & Ross-Hamid, 2012). At their first clinic appointment, women completed the EDS[1] and the anxiety subscale of HADS (HADS-A) and were asked to predict how they might be feeling in about 2 weeks' time. They were interviewed by telephone 2 weeks later and again completed the EDS and the HADS-A, and also answered questions about possible mood changes. Regardless of which cut-off scores on the EDS or HADS-A were used to define 'high' scorers, approximately 50% of women scoring 'high' at their first appointment on either measure no longer scored 'high' 2 weeks later. Common reasons given for their mood improvement included reduced morning sickness, reassuring results from routine tests (e.g. ultrasounds), fear of miscarriage subsiding, and a sense of reassurance following their hospital visit. Many were accurate in predicting at their first appointment that they would be feeling better soon. Referring women to specialist mental health services based on just one administration of these measures would obviously result in a large number of unnecessary referrals. The authors argue that when women score 'high' on a self-report scale, enquiring as to why this is the case and about whether the woman expects to feel differently in a

---

1. The reference to the EDS (Edinburgh Depression Scale) rather than the EPDS is an acronym that the authors of the scale do not now endorse. However, the EPDS may, when appropriate, be referred to as the Edinburgh Perinatal Depression Scale but always with the EPDS acronym and reference to the original publication in the *British Journal of Psychiatry*.

few weeks time, together with a second administration of the measures, is good practice, unless there are clinical reasons to do otherwise. It could also be argued that having mothers' low mood recognised and validated is in itself therapeutic.

Other antenatal prediction measures

Measures specifically designed to detect vulnerability factors may also prove effective in predicting depression. Several researchers have developed specific predictive measures, with differing claims of success. Elliott *et al* (1988) developed one of the earliest of these in a study of the prevention of postnatal depression.

In Manchester, UK, Appleby and colleagues (Appleby *et al*, 1994; Warner *et al*, 1997) developed a 10-item questionnaire based on psychosocial risk factors at 36 weeks. However, although antenatal scores on this questionnaire correlated significantly with EPDS scores at 8 weeks after birth, the questionnaire failed to discriminate between women who later did or did not develop depression according to psychiatric criteria. The team had more success using the 14-item Maternal Attitudes Questionnaire (MAQ), based on cognitions relating to role change, expectations of motherhood and expectations of the self as a mother. Maternal Attitudes Questionnaire scores correlated highly with scores on both the EPDS and the CIS (Warner *et al*, 1997).

In Reading, UK, Cooper *et al* (1996) tested a predictive index on a large sample of 5000 women who had completed an EPDS in the last trimester of pregnancy, and compared the results with the mental state of the women at 6–8 weeks postpartum. The authors claim that their index offers a system for the prediction of postpartum depression that could be of use in both research and clinical practice.

In a Danish study, Nielsen Forman *et al* (2000) gave an antenatal questionnaire on history of psychiatric disease, psychological distress and social support to 528 women during pregnancy and compared the results with EPDS scores at 4 months after delivery. They claimed that 1 in 3 women who have psychological distress in late pregnancy with perceived social isolation will develop postpartum depression. Similarly, Webster *et al* (2000) claimed improved recognition of women at risk of postnatal depression by using an 'objective, psychosocial assessment' (the Maternity Social Support Scale, MSSS) to screen 901 women antenatally in a hospital-based study in Queensland, Australia.

The overall picture emerging from antenatal screening for postnatal depression suggests that it is indeed helpful to ask women about their emotional state during pregnancy. As Green & Murray (1994) pointed out, organisationally, the antenatal care setting in the UK provides ideal opportunities for mass screening: most women attend a hospital clinic at least twice, see their midwife regularly and make several visits to their family doctor. However, the wide-scale implications must be carefully considered before deciding on routine screening. As with postnatal depression, organisational problems arise after screening. Who decides whether the woman should be further assessed and by whom? What treatment should she receive and who will administer this and supervise her care? For pregnant women with severe depression, do the benefits of antidepressants outweigh the risks? Not prescribing antidepressants for a woman with severe depression is potentially dangerous and can lead to suicide or infanticide. Advice on the risks of drugs is available from pharmacists or the UK Teratology Information Service (www.uktis.org). Referral to mental health services may be required, ideally to a specialist perinatal mental health service.

Identifying pregnant women at risk of developing puerperal psychosis

A most important task for midwives is not just to screen for current antenatal depression but also to identify women at high risk of developing puerperal psychosis. These are women with a history of psychosis, for whom there is at least a 1 in 4 risk of developing further psychosis. Also at risk are women with a family or personal history of severe depression, in particular manic or bipolar depression or a family history of puerperal psychosis.

It was pointed out by in *The Confidential Enquiries into Maternal Deaths in the United Kingdom* (Oates, 2001) that women with a history of severe mental disorder are often incorrectly categorised as having previous postnatal depression. This may lead to underestimation of the likely severity of a recurrence.

It is for this reason that simply administering the EPDS routinely at the booking-in clinical is not recommended. Rather, specific and sensitive inquiry should be made about psychiatric history. In particular, if the woman says that she had postnatal depression following a previous birth, the severity of the episode must be ascertained. As Oates (2001) points out:

> 'Most women who have experienced a previous severe postpartum mental illness will be concerned about future recurrence. All those involved, midwives, obstetricians, GPs and psychiatrists need to acquire knowledge of the high risk of recurrence, and to know that women with early onset conditions can quickly move from appearing to be merely anxious and depressed to being psychotic and suicidal within a few days. They also need to know that being mentally well during pregnancy does not necessarily reduce the risk of recurrence following delivery.
>
> Psychiatric, midwifery and obstetric staff need to communicate with each other and with the GP verbally and in writing about the care of women during pregnancy who are at risk of a postpartum mental illness.' (p. 186)

Conclusions from EPDS screening research

The EPDS is clearly being used in many ways and in many different contexts throughout the world. Research suggests that its use by health professionals can help them to identify both postnatal and antenatal depression. There are those who rightly criticise an oversystematised regime. In an article entitled 'Let's trust our instincts', Barker (1998) pointed out that health professionals should be encouraged to use their experience, insight and intuition, rather than relying on predetermined formulae to assess the well-being of their patients. However, as Taylor (1998) observed, 'relying on Walter Barker's somewhat sentimental ideas of intuition merely assists the de-skilling process that he says he is trying to prevent' (p. 427).

Clinical psychologists Angela Leviston and Maria Downs argue that instinct is not enough, maintaining that if used properly the scale can enhance clinical practice (Leviston & Downs, 1999). Most clinical studies have concluded that the majority of women readily accept routine use of the EPDS. However, it is important to remember that all were confidential research projects or sensitive clinical studies. Women's willingness to disclose personal information will, of course, be influenced by their perception of how that information will be used and who will have access to it. This point cannot be overemphasised. As Elliott & Leverton (2000) cogently point out in a review article:

> 'The EPDS is clearly not a magic wand to be distributed for compulsory use without training. Alone it is just a piece of paper, a checklist. Combined with training in prevention, detection and treatment, however, it becomes an important part of an effective programme.' (p. 303)

CHAPTER 5

Humanistic and person-centred interventions in perinatal depression

Maternal depression not only affects the quality of a woman's own life and experience of mothering, but can cast a long shadow on her whole family. Her reduced sensitivity may have adverse effects on her infant's emotional and cognitive development, and her other children may also be affected. For partnered women, increased irritability and loss of affectionate responsiveness may affect the couple's relationship or even lead to the break up of the family. Fathers may also have depression. Developing and practising preventive and therapeutic measures is both cost-effective and humane, and the importance of targeting scarce resources is increasingly acknowledged. In this chapter we examine innovative research in many parts of the world with implications for clinical practice.

The Edinburgh counselling intervention

The Edinburgh counselling intervention (Holden *et al*, 1989) gave health visitors a key role in finding practical ways of helping women with depression in a randomised controlled trial. Health visitors, who are qualified health professionals and part of the primary care team, provide a preventive health service. At the time of our research, most health visitors visited all women 10 days after childbirth, followed by regular assessments at home or clinic. They were thus in a key position to pick up problems and provide a link between a woman and her doctor and other services.

Seventeen health visitors in Edinburgh and Livingston (Scotland) were given brief training based on Rogerian non-directive (person-centred) counselling, using videos, case discussion, role-playing and written information about counselling, postnatal depression and how to administer the EPDS. They were asked to pay eight extra weekly 'listening' visits to women in their case-load who had been identified as having depression. Women who had scored 12 or above on the EPDS 6 weeks after giving birth were assessed for depression during a home visit about 3 months after the birth by a research psychiatrist using the CIS (Goldberg *et al*, 1970), with the diagnosis of depression derived from the RDC (Spitzer *et al*, 1978).

Women with depression were randomly allocated to the treatment group or to a control group that received routine primary care.

Health visitors were only informed of women in the treatment group, who received the weekly visits in their own home, when they were encouraged to talk about their feelings; questions about baby care were to be discussed separately. The health visitors were asked to counsel only those women referred to them. The research psychiatrist, who was given no information regarding the group to which each woman had been allocated, reassessed the women at home after 3 months.

In total, 50 women with postnatal depression completed the trial: 27 in the treatment group and 23 controls. Of the 27 counselled women, 18 showed no depression at the second interview, whereas only 9 of the 23 women who had received routine treatment had recovered. The percentages of recovered women in the treatment and control groups were 69% and 38% respectively. The difference, 32%, had a 95% confidence interval of 5–58%. The chi-squared statistic was 5.06, with one degree of freedom and an associated P-value of 0.03.

She just listened

'When my health visitor came at first I didn't much like her. She asked a lot of questions and was telling me what to do. I thought she meant I was doing things wrong. But when she came for the depression, she was completely different. I talked to her about how I felt and she just listened. When you talk about something it helps you sort things out, lets you see how small they are. Now I could tell her anything at all.' (Tape-recorded interview with a counselled woman; Holden, 1988)

We concluded that giving health visitors information about postnatal depression and instructions in using the EPDS and non-directive counselling could have a positive impact on the lives of women with postnatal depression. Confiding their feelings to their health visitor during counselling significantly reduced depressive symptoms. There were also other positive effects; in tape-recorded interviews at 10–12 months postnatal, many counselled women reported beneficial effects on their relationship with their partner and changes in their perception of the health visitor's role. Counselled women tended to view the health visitor as being there for them as well as for the baby, whereas women in the control group were less likely to see their health visitor as someone in whom they would be willing to confide (Holden, 1988).

Counselled women who still had depression after the intervention nevertheless benefited, as was demonstrated by their subsequent help-seeking behaviour. Of the non-recovered counselled women, 75% sought medical help, compared with only 13% of non-recovered controls. The attention of their health visitor may have encouraged counselled women to view their depression as a legitimate reason to consult, and having their depression validated may also have increased adherence to treatment.

However, it was disappointing that although their family doctors were informed of all women who still had depression after the trial, they did not offer help unless the woman herself sought it.

Once the study was under way we experienced surprisingly few problems, considering the considerable changes being made to normal practice. The health visitors had all 'opted in' and were enthusiastic about their part in the research, and weekly support meetings served to diffuse any anxieties. On recent enquiry, Edinburgh health visitors are still using EPDS screening and offering listening visits to women with postnatal depression.

Extending research findings into clinical practice

A large three-centre trial of health visitor training for postnatal depression was undertaken in London, Edinburgh and Stoke-on-Trent (Gerrard *et al*, 1994). The aim was to share what had been learned about the prevention, identification and treatment of postnatal depression and to give health visitors the opportunity to decide which aspects to adopt in their own work. Training included use of the EPDS and information about empathic listening and prevention, derived from our counselling study (Holden *et al*, 1989), with the inclusion of preventive measures derived from the study by Elliott *et al* (1988). The health visitors were encouraged to develop strategies based on local resources and to visit women in late pregnancy, to inform them about the study and about the possibility of depression. As some of the health visitors expressed concern at being asked to act as 'counsellors' without having received psychotherapeutic training, we changed the name of the intervention to 'listening visits'.

A comparison of women's EPDS scores at 6 months postnatal before and after training showed that participation in the programme enabled the health visitors to positively influence the emotional well-being of postnatal women, evidenced by a highly significant reduction in mean EPDS scores and in the numbers of women who scored above threshold (Gerrard *et al*, 1994; Elliott *et al*, 2001).

During this study, however, it was clear that referral pathways need to be clarified. In Edinburgh, health visitors could contact a community psychiatric nurse directly, who would accompany them on a home visit to women about whom they were concerned, with a view to further referral if required. In Stoke-on Trent, women could be referred directly to the Charles Street Parent and Baby Day Unit (Cox *et al*, 1993). In London, however, there was no pre-existing referral system and so a specialist psychiatrist was appointed.

The Cambridge intervention trials

Because of a mounting body of evidence of the adverse effects of maternal depression on infants' cognitive and emotional development,

Cooper & Murray (1997) embarked on a trial comparing three different psychosocial interventions administered by either a health visitor or a trained psychotherapist. As in our own counselling intervention (Holden *et al*, 1989), the health visitors and therapists had no responsibility for assessment or treatment decisions. Women in the Cambridge study were assessed for depression using a preliminary postal EPDS (scored by researchers) followed by a standardised psychiatric interview.

The four randomly assigned conditions were: non-directive counselling; cognitive–behavioural therapy (CBT) directed at problems of infant management such as feeding and sleeping; brief dynamic psychotherapy centred on the mother–infant relationship; and routine primary care. The EPDS and psychiatric interview were used to measure recovery from depression; effects on mother–infant interactions were assessed by videotaped interactions. Cooper & Murray (1997) reported a significant effect from all three brief interventions on speed of recovery from depression and on the quality of infants' attachment to recovered mothers. Early remission from depression, itself significantly related to receiving treatment, was associated with a reduced rate of insecure attachments. Importantly, there were no differences in outcome between either the type of intervention or whether the intervention was delivered by a trained psychotherapist or by a health visitor.

This led to a further intervention trial in which all Cambridge health visitors were taught to use a combination of counselling and cognitive–behavioural interventions at home-based visits, using the EPDS to assess depression and monitor recovery (Cooper & Murray, 1997; Murray *et al*, 2003). Levels of dysphoria and mothers' reports of relationship problems with their infants improved significantly compared with the control group, who received only routine treatment. The authors claimed that results from both of these studies show that health visitors who have been trained in the use of the EPDS and in the management and detection of postnatal depression can provide help that is both effective and acceptable to mothers, and also suggest that: 'it may be possible to interrupt potentially difficult cycles of interaction between mother and infant and thus prevent some of the adverse outcomes associated with postnatal depression' (Seeley *et al*, 1996).

The Ponder Trial

More recently, a large body of research into perinatal depression in the community has been undertaken in 101 general practices in England. In one aspect of the study, researchers, led by Jane Morrell of the University of Huddersfield, assessed the costs, effectiveness and broad impact of a randomised trial of two health visitor psychological interventions for postnatal depression. Over 4000 mothers were approached to receive either a cognitive–behavioural or a person-centred approach from specially trained health visitors, or to receive usual health visitor care (Morrell *et al*, 2009).

Health visitors in the intervention group were trained to identify depressive symptoms and to use clinical assessment skills to assess a mother's mood, including suicidal thoughts. They were also trained to deliver cognitive–behavioural or person-centred sessions for an hour per week for up to 8 weeks. Validated scales were used to assess depressive symptoms and participants were followed up for 18 months and assessed every 6 months using a postal questionnaire. The researchers found both approaches to be equally beneficial in reducing depressive symptoms compared with usual health visitor care (Morrell *et al*, 2009).

Following these encouraging findings, the investigators obtained funding for similar research in other areas. Sadly, Brugha *et al* (2011) reported that:

'When the research team set out to repeat and further develop this research they were unable to make sufficient progress because in most parts of England there has been a substantial reduction in the number of health visitors funded by the NHS. Mothers were fortunate if they received just one home visit from a health visitor. Health visitors were unable to take time off to undergo the extra training in assessment of depression and psychologically supportive approaches.'

This was indeed a cause for concern, as it is clear from this study and from our own research that health visitors are ideally qualified to take on this important work and are very willing to do so if they are enabled by funding. According to Cheryll Adams, Founding Director of the Institute of Health Visiting, the present government is taking the shortages very seriously and is committed to increase the number of health visitors by 50% by 2015. This work now has strong backing from the Department of Health (Department of Health, 2012), and the Institute of Health Visiting has recently been awarded the contract to train health visitors to cascade postnatal depression training across England (C. Adams, personal communication, 2013).

It is encouraging to learn that nurses in other countries have also risen to the challenge of helping mothers with depression using listening techniques.

Health visitor counselling in Sweden

Wickberg & Hwang (1996*b*) conducted a randomised trial of non-directive counselling based on our original study. They identified a sample of 57 women with depression using EPDS screening at 8 and 12 weeks and the Montgomery–Åsberg Depression Rating Scale (MADRS) and DSM-III-R at about 13 weeks postpartum. Forty-one women agreed to participate and were randomly allocated to counselling or a control group. Those in the counselling group received 6 weekly counselling visits by the child health clinic nurse and the control group received routine primary care. Of the 15 women with major depression in the counselling group, 12 (80%) were fully recovered after the intervention, compared with only 4 (25%) of the

16 women with major depression in the control group. As a result of this study the Swedish National Council for Medical Research recommended the implementation of postnatal screening and intervention throughout Sweden (C. Adams, personal communication, 2013). Almost all child healthcare centres have a consultant psychologist, who will train and offer regular supervision to staff.

Public health nurse counselling in Norway

In a controlled study by Glavin and colleagues (2010) in Oslo, public health nurses were trained to identify postpartum depression and provide supportive counselling. The EPDS was administered pre-test at 6 weeks and again at 3 and 6 months postnatal. Post-test scores in the experimental group decreased significantly compared with the comparison group at both 3 and 6 months. The authors concluded that non-directive counselling provided by public health nurses is an effective treatment method for postpartum depression.

Counselling in Australia

Milgrom *et al* (2011) conducted a trial in a primary care setting and a psychology clinic in Melbourne. Following EPDS screening, 68 women were randomised between treatment groups comparing management by GPs alone with adjunctive counselling, based on CBT, delivered by either postnatal nurses or psychologists. They found that all three treatment conditions were accompanied by significant reductions in depressive symptoms and that mean post-study BDI-II scores were similar between groups. Adherence was high in all three groups and women rated the treatments as highly effective. The authors suggest that GP management of postnatal depression when augmented by a CBT-counselling package may be successful in reducing depressive symptoms in more patients compared with GP management alone. However, they also reported relatively low rates of referral and treatment uptake, suggesting that help-seeking remains an issue for many women with postnatal depression, consistent with previous research, including our own.

Listening visits in Iowa, USA

It is not always necessary for a trial of treatment to be randomised in order to show its practicability within a given population. Segre and colleagues (2010) evaluated the effectiveness of listening visits with 19 women with depression from low-income backgrounds who were taking part in a Healthy Start programme. Healthy Start has home visitors who fulfil a similar role to UK health visitors. Importantly, they have a pre-existing rapport with their patients and are in an ideal position to provide a depression treatment such as listening visits. The home visitors attended perinatal workshops and received training from a listening visit specialist health visitor from the UK. The intervention was well accepted by the women, who showed significant improvements in the severity of their depression. They also reported significant improvement in life satisfaction including measures of how they were getting on at home, at work and with other people. This was a small-group study without controls and diagnostic assessments were not masked to condition. Nevertheless, this innovative real-life study showed that listening visits can help fill the gap in services for women who may not otherwise receive help. The authors are currently conducting a larger randomised controlled trial.

Comparing antidepressants with cognitive–behavioural counselling

Appleby et al's (1997) trial compared the antidepressant drug fluoxetine and cognitive–behavioural counselling in Manchester, UK. Sixty-one women with suspected depression 6–8 weeks after childbirth were randomly assigned to one of four treatment groups to receive a combination of fluoxetine or placebo, plus either one or six sessions of counselling. Counselling was delivered by health visitors who had received brief training.

Highly significant improvement was seen in all four treatment groups, the fluoxetine group showing significantly greater improvement than those receiving placebo. The authors concluded that both fluoxetine and cognitive–behavioural counselling are effective treatments for women with postnatal depression who do not have psychosis and that the women might therefore themselves make the choice of treatment. However, as the study also showed, many postnatal women are reluctant to take drug therapy. It could be an important task for a health professional to explain the effects and benefits of antidepressants and to encourage adherence to medication.

The RESPOND trial

A large study in Bristol, London and Manchester attempted to compare early treatment with antidepressants, general supportive care and non-directive counselling (listening visits) by specially trained research health visitors (Sharp et al, 2010). A total of 254 women who fulfilled ICD-10 criteria for major depression were recruited and randomly allocated. The authors found that antidepressants were clearly superior to general supportive care in reducing symptoms after 4 weeks (measured by EPDS scores), but it proved difficult to compare outcomes from antidepressant therapy with those from listening visits, as many of the women allocated to the counselled group also received antidepressants from their family doctor, and the counselling started 4 weeks later than the medication.

As the medication was started immediately but the counselling did not start for another 4 weeks, it seems hardly surprising that there was a benefit of medication over counselling after 4 weeks. This study does illustrate, however, the difficulties inherent in clinical practice research. Interestingly, qualitative interviews with women revealed:

> 'a preference for listening visits but an acceptance that antidepressants might be necessary. They wished to be reassured that their GP and [health visitor] were offering continuity of care focusing on their particular set of circumstances. Interviews with GPs and [health visitors] revealed lack of collaboration in managing care for women with [postnatal depression]; neither professional group was willing to assume responsibility' (Sharp et al, 2010).

Interpersonal psychotherapy

In Melbourne, Milgrom and colleagues (1999) reported positive outcomes from a small pilot study comparing different psychotherapeutic approaches with women with postnatal depression in a hospital setting. Women participated in groups led by two trained psychotherapists using a cognitive–behavioural approach based on work by Lewinsohn et al (1984) and Olioff (1991).

O'Hara et al (2000) described a randomised controlled trial of interpersonal psychotherapy with women in North America meeting DSM-IV criteria for postnatal depression. Of those who received 12 sessions of interpersonal psychotherapy, 60% showed a significant improvement compared with only 20% of waiting-list controls. Therapy was, however, conducted by 10 trained psychotherapists, who each read specified manuals and received 40 hours of didactic lectures and training; such an expensive intervention would be difficult to replicate in primary care.

Preventive antenatal interventions

Some researchers have directed their attention to interventions aimed at preventing depression after childbirth, with varying success. Non-pharmacological interventions that have been shown to be effective in postnatal depression (e.g. listening visits, cognitive therapy) have also been evaluated for their effectiveness in treating depression in pregnancy. In a large prospective study in which the EPDS was administered by midwives, Green & Murray (1994) concluded that the women at greatest risk of continuing depression were those with poor marital relationships and no one to talk to. The researchers were encouraged to find that midwives were responding with significantly more home visits to such women.

In a controlled study of enhanced midwifery practice involving over 2000 women, 36 general practice clusters in the West Midlands (UK) were randomly allocated to intervention or routine treatment. Midwives in both groups attended a study day and those in the intervention group received extra training in the new model of care. Symptom checklists and the EPDS were used to identify individual needs and guidelines were given to the midwives for the management of these needs. Care was extended to 28 days, with a discharge consultation at 10–12 weeks. The redesigned community postnatal care package was associated with improved mental health outcomes for the intervention group, including reduction in EPDS scores (MacArthur et al, 2002). The researchers concluded that 'this study suggests an extended role for midwives in the emotional well-being of women in their care and the importance of including midwives in developing a local perinatal mental health strategy, as recommended by the Royal College of Psychiatrists'.

In a controlled trial in the USA, Spinelli & Endicott (2003) compared a group receiving interpersonal psychotherapy for antenatal depression with a parenting education control programme. Of the women treated with interpersonal psychotherapy, 60% recovered from their depression and there was also a significant correlation between maternal mood and mother–infant interaction. Spinelli & Endicott concluded that interpersonal psychotherapy should be a first-line treatment in the hierarchy of treatment for antepartum depression.

In 1999, Steinberg & Bellavance conducted a longitudinal prospective study with pregnant women, 91 of whom had depression and 45 who did not; the study continued over 6 months into the postnatal period. They used individual psychotherapy, combining strategies from interpersonal and cognitive–behavioural psychotherapy and/or marital interventions and pharmacology. Although depressive symptoms (measured by the EPDS and the HRSD) in the index group generally improved by the second to third month of treatment, marital discord and child care stress levels did not. The authors concluded that although short-term interventions are a cost-effective way of dealing with depression, 'creative solutions are required to extend treatment sufficiently to address couple conflicts and facilitate the transition to parenthood'.

Antenatal support and information groups

Some antenatal interventions have been based on ideas that could be incorporated into existing systems of antenatal classes and/or postnatal support groups. Two early studies are still worthy of note. First, over 40 years ago Gordan & Gordan (1960) added two 40-minute sessions to traditional antenatal classes, in which women and their partners were advised to seek information and practical help, to make friends with couples experienced in childcare, to avoid moving house, to get plenty of rest, to discuss plans and worries, to cut down unnecessary activities and to arrange babysitters. They reported that women who were encouraged during pregnancy to confide in their husbands and enlist their practical help not only received more help, but were also less likely to develop depression.

Shereshefsky & Lockman (1973) showed that the marital relationships of women who received individual antenatal counselling about the possible effect of childbirth on their relationship remained stable, whereas those in a control group had deteriorated by 6 months postpartum.

Elliott and colleagues (1988) invited pregnant women identified as being vulnerable to developing depression, to informal locally based antenatal groups designed to give professional support and information about coping strategies during pregnancy and after the birth. The groups also provided the opportunity to meet other women and develop peer-group support. Although attendance among second-time mothers was low and the numbers in this study were small, at 6 months after delivery the invited first-time mothers showed only half the prevalence of postnatal depression found in non-invited mothers.

Other preventive interventions have proved less than successful. In Adelaide, Australia, Stamp *et al* (1995) invited women identified as vulnerable using a modified antenatal screening questionnaire to support groups that met during pregnancy and continued postnatally. The control group had no intervention. Sadly, attendance at their groups was low and the intervention did not reduce postnatal depression. They concluded that using groups separate from the standard antenatal classes may have affected attendance, and that more research is required into ways of reaching and supporting women who may develop depression.

Brugha *et al* (2000) in Leicester, England, conducted a larger trial. Their programme 'Preparing for Parenthood' was designed to increase social support and improve problem-solving skills. Of the 1300 pregnant women originally screened, outcome data were obtained from 190 women at 3 months after childbirth. Of the women in the intervention group, 45% had attended sufficient sessions to be likely to benefit. However, this intervention was not effective in preventing postnatal depression, as attenders derived no more benefit than non-attenders. These authors also concluded that further research is needed.

Zlotnick and colleagues (2001) in the USA were more successful. They found that a four-session interpersonal-therapy-oriented group intervention was effective in preventing the occurrence of major depression in a group of financially disadvantaged women. Pregnant women who had at least one risk factor for postnatal depression were randomly assigned to a four-session group intervention or to a treatment-as-usual condition. Of 37 women, 35 completed the study; structured diagnostic interviews were used to assess for postnatal major depression. Within 3 months after they gave birth, 6 of the 18 women in the treatment-as-usual condition had developed postpartum major depression, compared with none of the 17 women in the intervention condition. The authors concluded that: 'Our finding of the significant efficacy of the group intervention differs from the results of previous studies possibly because of the higher compliance rate in the current study.'

In Norway, Kozinszky *et al* (2012) evaluated the effectiveness of a brief preventive randomised group intervention and studied the effect of this on social and psychological risk factors. The intervention appeared to significantly reduce the risk of depression, as defined by Leverton Questionnaire total scores. They concluded that 'a brief preventive antepartum group intervention focusing on psychoeducation, stress management, improving coping mechanisms, and the development of social support can be effective in reducing postpartum depressive symptomatology'.

Infant massage and postnatal support

Onozawa *et al* (2001) in London tried regular infant massage classes to reduce maternal depression and improve the quality of mother–infant interaction. Thirty-four mothers with first-time depression were randomly allocated either to an infant massage class and support group or to a control support group for five weekly sessions from about 9 weeks postnatal. EPDS scores fell in both groups, but significant improvements in mother–infant interaction (assessed by videotape ratings) were seen only in the massage group. The sample size was small and the authors were unable to distinguish which aspects of the massage class contributed to the benefit, but concluded that learning infant massage is an effective way of facilitating mother–infant interaction.

Massage therapy for expectant mothers

Field (1998) designed a 6-week antenatal programme to determine whether massage therapy would facilitate adherence to psychotherapy. Pregnant women with depression were randomly assigned either to a group who received only group psychotherapy or to one who received both group psychotherapy and massage. The process appeared to be effective for both groups. The group who received psychotherapy plus massage attended more sessions on average and a greater percentage completed the course. This group also showed a greater decrease on depression and anxiety scores and a decrease in cortisol levels, showing the facilitative effects of massage therapy on group interpersonal psychotherapy for reducing prenatal depression.

Postnatal interventions involving partners

Some researchers have explored the possibility of enlisting the support of fathers either in helping mothers with postnatal depression or in a preventive role. In a small controlled study in British Columbia, Misri and colleagues (2000) conducted a trial of partner support with 29 women who met DSM-IV criteria for postnatal depression. The support group consisted of women and their partners, with only women in the control group. The participants in both groups were each seen for seven psychoeducational visits; partners in the support group took part in four of the seven visits. Depressive symptoms in the index group women decreased significantly, as measured by the GHQ and the EPDS. The authors concluded that partner support has a measurable effect on women experiencing postnatal depression. Interestingly, when only the women (and not their partners) received the intervention the general health of the women's partners deteriorated. This effect was not found where the men were included in the intervention.

In Sydney, Australia, Barnett *et al* described a group programme for distressed postnatal women and their partners consisting of eight sessions, including one session for the couple. Psychotherapeutic and cognitive–behavioural strategies were used to help the women deal with concerns such as their anxieties and feelings towards their partners, their own mothers and their infants. The programme also encouraged the men to provide emotional and practical support to their partner. Interestingly, although the programme was successful over time in reducing maternal distress and increasing mothers' self-esteem, about half of the men showed elevated levels of distress (Morgan *et al*, 1997).

Antenatal interventions involving partners

Women who had taken part in our original counselling study, especially those in the non-intervention group, described the inadequacy of antenatal information for both parents.

> 'They should tell you when you're pregnant what to expect. And they should tell the men. If men understood more, they'd be able to help more rather than just saying: "will you shut up and stop crying, go upstairs if you want to cry"'.
> (Tape-recorded interview with a control group woman; Holden *et al*, 1989)

A controlled trial of a brief antenatal group intervention with mothers and fathers, addressing infant behaviour and couple-relationship management, found dramatically lower instances of depression and/or anxiety among women who had attended the couples-group session than among those who had met with a health visitor at home (Fisher *et al*, 2010).

An inexpensive antenatal intervention in the USA consisting of one prenatal session in separate men/women groups which focused on psychosocial issues related to becoming first-time parents was associated with reduced distress in some mothers at 6 weeks postpartum. The key factor seemed to be the women's perception of an increased level of awareness in the men as to how they were experiencing the early weeks after the birth (Matthey *et al*, 2004). In a more recent Australian controlled trial, home visiting nurses provided information, psychosocial support and health-promoting activities for families in an area of socioeconomic disadvantage in Western Sydney. Intervention mothers had a higher rate of unassisted vaginal births than the general population, and at 4–6 weeks postnatally reported better general health and felt significantly more enabled to cope with and understand their baby and to care for themselves and their baby than control mothers (Kemp *et al*, 2013).

Partners as massage therapists for women with antenatal depression

An interesting study by Field and colleagues (2004) looked at the effectiveness of massage in helping pregnant women who already had major depression. The women were either provided with 12 weeks of twice-a-week massage therapy delivered by their partner or received standard treatment. The massage group not only had reduced depression and cortisol by the end of the treatment period, but also had reduced depression in the postnatal period. Their newborns were also less likely to be born prematurely and of low birthweight, had lower cortisol levels and performed better on the Neonatal Behavioral Assessment Scale (NBAS) habituation, orientation and motor subscales. Scores on a relationship questionnaire improved more for both the women and their partners in the massage group. Both mood states and relationships improved when pregnant women with depression were massaged by their partner. There were also positive effects on their infants.

Interventions for fathers

As Wee *et al* (2011) pointed out, the study of paternal depression is relatively new, and there have so far been few interventions directed towards this important group. One notable exception is the work of Svend Madsen in Denmark, who has conducted extensive research into fatherhood and male postnatal depression. His work focuses on the development of male-sensitive communication with fathers in existing health services, with research directed to creating and implementing male- and father-specific methods in psychotherapy. He also oversees a well-frequented website for fathers (www.european-fatherhood.com).

Developing specific interventions to help fathers with depression is obviously long overdue, but many men are reluctant to present themselves as needing help. Routinely assessing men's mental health in the perinatal period could lead to the identification of treatable problems that would otherwise go undetected – benefiting not only the fathers themselves but the whole family. It may also help fathers to feel included in healthcare provision. Six months after the intervention in our original counselling study was completed, Holden visited all the participating women at home and conducted tape-recoded interviews about their experience of depression. Fortuitously, partners were present at several of the interviews and most were eager to participate. One father said: 'that woman (the health visitor) came every week to see her, but nobody cares about how

I'm feeling' (Holden, 1988). When embarking on a programme of listening visits with a mother with depression, it would perhaps be advantageous to include a session for the father either on his own or with his partner, to be decided by the couple's preference.

Day hospital care

North Staffordshire in the UK was uniquely favoured by having a psychiatric day unit for mothers with postnatal depression and their babies (Cox *et al*, 1993). The atmosphere was informal and welcoming, the underlying philosophy being that many cases are likely to have psychosocial origins. Members of the multidisciplinary team were trained in non-directive counselling and also familiarity with the range of antidepressant medication. Cognitive therapy was available from a clinical psychologist. Activities included yoga, meditation, individual and group therapy, relaxation, a stress-management group, assertiveness training and creative therapy (including art and role-play).

Boath *et al* (1999, 2003) compared 30 women treated at the North Staffordshire facility with 30 women who received routine primary care. Clinical, marital and social adjustment were measured using the EPDS, the CIS, the anxiety subscale of the HRSD, the Dyadic Adjustment Scale (DAS) and the Work Leisure and Family Life Questionnaire (WLFLQ). At baseline the groups were similar, but there were significant differences in outcome at 3- and 6-month follow-up for all measures except the DAS. Doctors and health visitors were informed of any women in the primary care treatment group who had depression and of the progress of the women in both groups. The team anticipated that:

> 'providing these professionals with a diagnosis would influence treatment and hence improve clinical outcome … our findings suggest that being told that a woman has postnatal depression does not in itself lead to effective treatment' (Boath *et al*, 1999: p. 150).

These findings echoed our own disappointment with the lack of doctor-initiated follow-up care provided to women who had taken part in our counselling study. As the authors point out, this may indicate a need to train doctors to screen for postnatal depression and how to treat it.

Caring for women with postnatal depression in rural areas

In a fascinating small study in Victoria, Australia, Craig and colleagues (2005) trained community health workers to deliver a 9-week cognitive–behavioural group programme to women with postnatal depression living in a rural setting. The programme was successful in leading to reduced EPDS and HADS scores, and reduction in symptoms was maintained at follow-up. The authors describe the many problems to be overcome in undertaking such a programme: lack of specialist mental health provision, fear of stigmatisation and distorted perceptions of postnatal depression among women themselves and the wider community, leading to difficulties in recruitment.

In areas where contact with health services is limited (and where women with depression may be reluctant to come forward), telephone or internet-based help may be a lifeline.

Telephone counselling

Thome & Alder (1999) claimed successful results from a randomised controlled trial of a telephone intervention in Iceland to reduce fatigue and its resulting distress symptoms in 78 mothers who reported having a behaviourally difficult infant 2–3 months of age. Simple telephone interventions could perhaps be further developed as part of health service provision.

In Canada, Dennis and colleagues (2009) conducted a randomised controlled trial in seven health regions across Ontario to evaluate the effectiveness of telephone-based peer support in the prevention of postnatal depression. Women in the treatment group received telephone-based peer support provided by a volunteer recruited from the community who had previously experienced and recovered from self-reported postnatal depression and attended a 4-hour training session. At 12 weeks, 14% of women in the intervention group and 25% in the control group had an EPDS score >12. Over 80% of women in the intervention group who received and evaluated the intervention were satisfied and would recommend this support to a friend. The researchers concluded that telephone-based peer support can be effective in preventing postnatal depression among women at high risk.

A perinatal and infant mental health service in Perth, Western Australia, report that their telephone support line for women in rural areas is increasing in demand year by year. Caroline Zanetti and her colleagues hope to extend their service to include face-to-face interactions using electronic media (e.g. Skype) with the caveat that: 'therapy should start with a face-to-face assessment of the woman's presentation and needs, as this will help create the necessary therapeutic alliance and mitigate risk' (C. Zanetti, personal communication, 2012).

The internet

Increasing use of the internet has introduced the possibility of innovations in both research and intervention, especially in remote areas. In Australia, Danaher *et al* (2012) designed an internet-based intervention using CBT. A controlled study of the Mum Mood Booster programme is underway.

The Norwegian Women's Public Health Association and the Regional Centre for Child and Adolescent Mental Health in Eastern and Southern Norway have set up what they describe as 'the world's first [...] interactive and individualised intervention for the prevention of postpartum depression' (Changetech, 2010). They aim to prepare parents for the birth, and to support the connection between mother and child during and after pregnancy. They will use individualised feedback and cognitive therapy to reduce symptoms of depression, and also to increase perceived social support for the mother. Fathers are invited to participate and will receive information about the importance of giving care and support to the mother during pregnancy and after birth. The Mamma Mia programmme was presented at the International Marcé Society Conference in 2010.

Another treatment programme is being developed by the University of Exeter and the parenting website Netmums, based on a pilot study in which partaking women showed significant improvements compared with those who continued their usual treatment. Women reported that they appreciated being able to take part in the course in their own time, online from home. The study will include online CBT and telephone sessions provided by a trained supporter. The researchers report that: 'this innovative approach to treatment has been created in response to the stigma that still surrounds postnatal depression, preventing many women from seeking help' (O'Mahen, 2012). They hope that this free programme will pave the way for future online treatments for depression.

Australia's online Post and Antenatal Depression Association (PANDA) has recently been rated as the worldwide website leader for mothers with a postnatal mental illness in an independent study by the University of Sussex (Moore & Ayers, 2011).

The internet has also been used to collect data. In a longitudinal study in Norway, the researchers, who aimed to explore possible predictors of postnatal depression, used internet-based questionnaires to collect data from 737 new mothers at 6 weeks, 3 months and 6 months postpartum. (Haga *et al*, 2012). Although it could perhaps be argued that women responding to an online survey may not be representative of the general population, this approach offers interesting possibilities.

Other ways of helping during the perinatal period

Many of the studies discussed in this chapter contain ideas and strategies that health professionals may be able to adapt in their own practice. There are, however, other simple ways of helping women during the perinatal period. Primary care workers are, for example, ideally placed to put women in touch with others in a similar situation and to encourage 'befriending' of newcomers or women who have perhaps been at work and do not know many other women in their locality.

Liaison with other agencies

Health professionals are usually familiar with other forms of help that may be available locally and encourage women to utilise them. In the UK, for example, one empowering scheme is Home-Start, a voluntary home-visiting programme with over 100 branches. Home-Start works closely with both statutory and voluntary agencies, and has paid organisers and secretaries, and volunteers who have been 'realistically recruited, carefully prepared, sensitively matched with only one or two families at a time, and meticulously supported' (Harrison, 1992). Volunteers offer friendship, support and practical help to young families experiencing difficulties for up to 2 years after the birth of their child, acting as a friend and confidant and helping to build self-confidence in using other services. Self-help groups can also increase mothers' self-confidence by giving them the opportunity to discuss shared experiences. The Meet-a-Mum Association (MAMA) offers informal home-based groups for mothers who feel isolated after the birth and also offers a supportive internet service.

In Australia, the excellent work of the Tresillian Family Centre is well known. In the UK, Crysis is a specialised association for parents whose babies cry excessively, with groups and telephone contacts. The Association for Postnatal Illness has had an important role in publicising postnatal depression and in helping individual women by giving them a telephone supporter. Women who have benefited from such help often go on to become volunteer helpers themselves. Alternative therapies such as relaxation, aromatherapy or art therapy may also be available locally.

Information

Routine contacts in health centre settings can provide opportunistic teaching and support sessions, and the waiting room is an ideal place for explanatory posters and leaflets. An updated list of information about facilities available in the area is also valuable. Pace (1992) described a health education library in general practice with 400 books in the waiting room for patients to 'dip into' or borrow. Books on mental health and childcare were the most popular. One recently published self-help book for mothers with depression is *Overcoming Postnatal Depression: A Five Areas Approach* (Williams *et al*, 2009).

There is clearly a wide range of ways in which perinatal women and their partners can be helped to enjoy this precious time with their new infant. As Boath & Henshaw (2001) cogently concluded:

'Based on the variable success of interventions...and the premise that postnatal depression results from a multitude of individual and contextual factors, it is feasible that no single intervention can treat all episodes of postnatal depression. Thus a multi-faceted, integrated approach, involving links between the formal and informal services that are currently available, collaboration between primary care professionals and community and secondary psychiatric staff, and patient education and involvement, that would allow women to choose the intervention(s) most relevant to their needs should be explored' (p. 243).

Conclusions

Much exciting and innovative work is being carried out worldwide, based on humanistic, person-centred approaches to helping women with perinatal distress. Strategies most likely to succeed are those that lead to empowerment and increased feelings of self-worth for the individual. However, long-term follow-up studies may be needed to demonstrate the true effectiveness of early interventions. Some perinatal healthcare staff (including health visitors and doctors) may wish to formalise their intervention skills training by undertaking a course accredited by a recognised organisation such as the Counselling and Psychotherapy Central Awarding Body.

CHAPTER 6

Screening and intervention services in the community

The consequences of maternal depression are costly not only on a personal level, but also in terms of health service resources, including money as well as personnel. It is important therefore that services should be relevant, targeted and research-based. The fact that women's contact with health professionals is at a peak around the time of childbirth provides an ideal opportunity for intervention and for ensuring that these contacts are used with maximum efficiency to meet the needs of individual women.

In this chapter we discuss the argument for introducing the EPDS in healthcare settings. Information was derived from research and from training groups of health professionals from different disciplines (including psychologists, psychiatrists family doctors, community psychiatric nurses, midwives and health visitors) for the introduction of postnatal depression initiatives. Discussions during training and post-training feedback added to our knowledge of the practical issues of administering the EPDS.

Following our original EPDS and counselling intervention research (Cox et al, 1987; Holden et al, 1989), training was requested by health authorities in England, Scotland, Northern Ireland and Ireland and many primary care trusts introduced routine EPDS screening and intervention programmes. In 2002, the SIGN Development Group carried out a survey of EPDS practice (Scottish Intercollegiate Guidelines Network, 2002). SIGN found that EPDS screening was undertaken routinely in all but one primary care trust area in Scotland. They recommended the use of the EPDS as a screening tool, but the document also pointed out that:

> 'the routine use of the EPDS carries significant implications associated with training, health visitor time for screening and intervention, and facilities in general practice and secondary care for treatment.' (p. 17)

The routine screening debate

It has been suggested that administering the EPDS with all postnatal women is both unnecessary and intrusive (Shakespeare, 2002), and that experienced health professionals who are in frequent contact with their patients should be able to detect depression without such an aid (Barker, 1998). In 2009, Paulden and colleagues evaluated several screening measures for postnatal depression (including the EPDS) to determine their value within the NHS. They concluded that although the major determinant of cost-effectiveness seems to be the potential additional costs of managing women incorrectly diagnosed with depression, the routine application of either postnatal or general depression questionnaires did not seem to be cost-effective compared with routine care only and 'do not currently satisfy the National Screening Committee's criteria for the adoption of a screening strategy as part of national health policy'.

In 1997, Whooley *et al* compared a two-question case-finding instrument with other depression measures in a veterans' clinic in San Francisco, USA. They concluded that it was a useful measure for detecting depression in primary care, having similar test characteristics to other case-finding instruments and being less time-consuming. In 2007, NICE issued clinical guidance on the management of antenatal and postnatal mental healthcare, recommending the use of the two Whooley questions as a routine screen for postnatal depression. They are:

1   'During the past month, have you often been bothered by feeling down, depressed or hopeless?'

2   'During the past month, have you often been bothered by little interest or pleasure in doing things?'

A third question should be considered if the woman answers 'yes' to either of the initial questions: 'Is this something you feel you need or want help with?'

When Hewitt *et al* conducted an analysis of postnatal depression screening as a National Institute for Health Research Health Technology Assessment in 2009, however, they found no evidence for these three questions in terms of validity, acceptability and clinical and cost-effectiveness in a postnatal population. On the other hand, they found that in the majority of studies:

> 'the EPDS was acceptable to women and healthcare professionals when women were forewarned of the process, when the EPDS was administered in the home, with due attention to training those administering the EPDS, with empathic skills of the health visitor and due consideration of positive responses to question 10 about self-harm.' (p. xii)

According to Gemmill and colleagues (2006), opinion on the utility of screening for postnatal depression remains mixed. Bodies such as the American Congress of Obstetricians and Gynecologists fully endorse the routine screening of postnatal women with the EPDS and health bodies in other countries have adopted similar policies after due weighing of the evidence. By contrast, the UK government considers that universal screening with the EPDS does not yet meet its statutory criteria. There remains a need for further controlled studies of perinatal depression, the validation of the EPDS in naturalistic, community settings as well as its comparison with standardised questions such as the Whooley questions.

Arguments for routine screening

Research consistently shows that even where contact between professionals and mothers is high, detection of postnatal depression is low. Failure to diagnose depression may be due to short appointments, a physical orientation of care and an emphasis on the baby's rather than the mother's well-being. During the first 6 weeks after the birth, postnatal depression may be hard to differentiate from the normal adjustment to the infant, but by the end of this period healthcare input normally lessens. In today's economic climate, regular home visits may be increasingly difficult to achieve.

Problems with routine screening

Shakespeare (2002) reported on an audit in Oxford, UK, studying the effectiveness of services delivered to postnatal women in 26 primary care practices. Health visitors who had been trained by a psychiatrist and a psychologist used routine EPDS screening at about 6–8 weeks and 8 months (Gerrard et al, 1994). Shakespeare found that only 66% of women were screened at 6–8 weeks and this dropped to 55% at 8 months. It was considered that workloads in deprived areas may be disproportionately high, presentation of the EPDS may differ from one practice to another, and resource and training issues were also identified.

Should nurses intervene in postnatal depression?

As Elliott (1994) pointed out, health visitors are not a treatment agency, although 'pressure of work often finds them operating a crisis intervention or treatment service' (p. 230). Mead et al (1997), who examined the potential and current role and training needs of nurses, found that although they are already involved in emotional healthcare with a variety of patient groups, this is not always acknowledged as mental health work. Corney (1980), who studied referrals to social workers by health visitors, found that they rarely referred patients with emotional or relationship problems, but tried to help them by providing social support and making frequent visits, sometimes several times a week. In cases of depression, the health visitor would become someone the patient could talk to, someone to be there when the patient cries. They would often encourage patients to express their feelings, but were sometimes anxious that they would 'get out of their depth'.

The results of community-based intervention trials indicate strongly that if health visitors are given adequate training and support, they can positively influence the outcome for women with perinatal depression (Holden et al, 1989; Gerrard et al, 1994; Seeley et al, 1996; Cooper & Murray, 1997; Elliott et al, 2000). Taylor (1989), Angeli & Grahame (1990), Cullinan

(1991) and Painter (1995) all reported that using the EPDS and supportive counselling led to increased identification and decreased symptoms among women with depression and also increased the confidence of the health visitors in caring for them.

Studies in other countries have examined ways in which primary care or hospital-based nurses can become involved with the evaluation of postnatal depression. In Sweden, Wickberg & Hwang (1996b) conducted a successful study of nurse counselling in Sweden, and Holt (1995) reported positively on EPDS identification by primary care nurses in New Zealand. Webster *et al* (2000), also in New Zealand, reported on midwives who compared the EPDS responses of European and Maori women; and Schaper *et al* (1994) examined the effectiveness of EPDS identification by midwives and doctors in Wisconsin, USA. In Australia, Stamp & Crowther (1994) looked at mothers' perceptions of midwives' care and attitudes; and in Japan, Suzuki (2001) described a midwife-led perinatal support system that emphasised the importance of ensuring that the views and feelings of women are acknowledged.

The need for training

Nurses in many countries are clearly involved in caring for the emotional needs of women with postnatal depression. It is, however, important both for the professionals and for the women they care for that the potential difficulties of such an extended role are clearly acknowledged by management. As Seeley (2001) remarked,

> 'the EPDS is only as good as the person using it. Where there is no, or inadequate training, individual health visitors will use it as best they can, but this may not be good enough' (p. 17).

The EPDS can be misused if it is administered without prior explanation by professionals who have not been trained in its use and without the full support of health managers and interdisciplinary colleagues. Recognition of the extra time needed, standardised training programmes and assurance that expert help and support from psychiatrists, psychologists and community psychiatric nurses are readily accessible are essential prerequisites for any postnatal depression programme to be successful.

Physicians' training in perinatal depression

When we first started our research in 1983, we asked a family doctor how women with postnatal depression were cared for in primary care. We were surprised to learn that, in his opinion, most doctors knew little about postnatal depression, which was not at that time included in the training of undergraduates. Most doctors learned about the condition only by being confronted with women with postnatal depression in their practice.

Small and colleagues in Australia compared the views of 134 undergraduate medical students about postnatal depression with those of 60 women who had themselves experienced it (Small *et al*, 1997). The women's and students' views differed markedly: students were more likely to view hormonal and biological factors and a 'tendency to depression' as being relevant, whereas the women identified a wide range of social, physical health and life-event factors as contributing to their depression. Fourth-year students tended to overestimate the prevalence of depression and sixth-year students to underestimate it. Both student groups underestimated the duration of depression compared with women's actual experiences. The authors concluded that medical students need to develop a broader understanding of maternal depression after the birth of a baby, and that women's own views of the experience can and should make an important contribution to medical teaching on this topic.

Aitken & Jacobson (1997), who sent a questionnaire to 173 psychiatrists and 350 GPs in the UK, found that these groups had a low level of awareness and knowledge of the EPDS, had little experience in its use and would not feel confident in giving advice on issues arising from its use by health visitors. Boath *et al*'s (1999) comparison of routine treatment with treatment at a parent and baby day unit revealed differences in clinical outcome that clearly demonstrate the need to provide training to all health professionals on how to detect and treat postnatal depression.

A shared framework of understanding

The term postnatal depression is often loosely used to describe a range of symptoms from tearfulness and emotional lability to the disconnection from reality of puerperal psychosis. Interpretation depends on both the user and the context. A psychiatrist, for example, may define minor depression in very different terms from those used by a woman experiencing it. To avoid misunderstandings and ensure that each woman receives individualised care, it is important that all professionals have a shared understanding of the range of severity and possible origins of the condition and of various intervention options, including psychological measures as well as medication (Holden, 1996).

The steering committee

'The EPDS is a short and simple tool, but its introduction into primary care is anything but simple. In its wake it carries widespread system change as well as a new philosophy.' (Elliott, 1994: p. 229)

Before starting a postnatal initiative, it is essential to set up an interdisciplinary steering committee with representatives from maternity, obstetric and psychiatric primary care services. The committee should produce recommendations on services and guidelines consistent with the services available in the locality. All services should be informed of the new programme and of decisions reached by the committee.

The need for clearly identified referral systems

Many cases of postnatal depression can be dealt with at the primary-care level, with monitoring by the family doctor and brief interventions by primary care staff. However, most of those who will be administering the EPDS are unlikely to have in-depth psychiatric knowledge. The health visitor or primary care nurse should not be expected to take sole responsibility for deciding, on the basis of a raised EPDS score, who has depression or who is suitable for an intervention. In the first instance, decisions should be made in collaboration with the family doctor.

Many of those who cannot be helped by simple measures do not need expensive psychiatric assessments, but do need longer or more specialist therapy. Some women will definitely require more intensive help. Those caring for perinatal women need to know where and how to refer, and they need to know that psychiatrists, psychologists and community psychiatric nurses are not only willing and able to accept referrals, but understand the special needs of this patient group.

Implications of scores on EPDS item 10, self-harm

In tape-recorded interviews conducted after the intervention in our counselling trial, many of the women confessed to having felt desperate during their depression:

> 'I've been sad and unhappy and miserable before, but never to the extent that I got with Thomas, to the point where I just didn't want to live any more.'

> 'If it hadn't been for the wee one, I'd definitely have jumped.' (Holden, 1988)

It is reassuring to know that the majority of women with a small infant are unlikely to act on such feelings. When Appleby (1991) retrospectively examined population data from England and Wales for 1973–1984, he found that the rate of suicide among women in the first postnatal year was only a sixth of that expected in a matched female population. However, *The Confidential Enquiries into Maternal Deaths in the United Kingdom* (Oates, 2001) found that, although rare (only 1 or 2 per 100000 maternities), death from suicide is the most common cause of maternal deaths. None of the women who died by suicide between 1997 and 1999 had been managed by a specialist perinatal mental health team, nor had any been admitted at any time to a mother and baby unit.

There is as yet little published evidence linking suicidal ideation and risk with responses to item 10 on the EPDS. However, one interesting community-based study found that an indication of thoughts of self-harm on the EPDS did not necessarily alert health professionals. In

Rochester, Minnesota, USA, where universal screening was implemented in all community postnatal care sites, some degree of suicidal ideation was noted on the EPDS by 48 women, but this was acknowledged in the medical records of only 10 women, including one who required immediate admission to hospital (Georgiopoulos *et al*, 2001).

In the large RESPOND trial in the UK, Howard *et al* found that 4% of 4150 women at about 6 weeks postpartum had suicidal ideation occurring sometimes or quite often and 9% reported any suicidal ideation. This is the only study to compare suicidal ideation with another measure of suicidality, the revised CIS (CIS-R). Responding 'yes, quite often' to item 10 was associated with affirming at least two CIS-R items on suicidality. However, a positive response to item 10 at 6 weeks was not associated with outcome on follow-up. The authors suggest that this probably reflects the fact that women in the RESPOND trial were treated for depression with either medication or psychotherapy (Howard *et al*, 2011).

A positive score on EPDS item 10 should always be taken seriously. In any screening programme a protocol for acting on a positive score on item 10 should be clearly defined. The response should be sensitively discussed and an extra visit arranged. For some women simply being able to talk about suicidal thoughts and having their feelings validated will diffuse the situation. In more serious cases, referral to psychiatric services may be appropriate. The woman should be assured that non-judgemental help is available and that if she continues to feel suicidal, she should immediately contact her health visitor or family doctor, or walk into the emergency clinic in a local psychiatric facility.

The need for specialist psychiatric services

In *The Confidential Enquiries into Maternal Deaths in the United Kingdom*, Oates wrote:

> 'there has been little improvement in the care for those suffering from severe mental illness in association with childbirth. The majority of women who suffer from these conditions still do not have access to mental health professionals with specialist knowledge and skills, nor to a mother-and-baby unit, should they require admission for puerperal psychosis' (Oates, 2001: p. 169).

For effective secondary prevention of impact on the child and family, during the postnatal period women should be seen more quickly than is possible in a typical secondary care psychology or psychotherapy service. Even when it has been decided that primary care staff will treat a woman with depression, problems may arise that are beyond the staff's range of knowledge. They are likely to encounter many ambiguous situations calling for complex decisions; for example, a woman may confide a history of intimate partner abuse, suicidal impulses or fears that she may abuse her child. Referral policy should be clear and simple.

In England and Wales, service provision recommendations are now contained in the *Guide for Commissioners of Perinatal Mental Health Services* (Joint Commisioning Panel for Mental Health, 2012). The guideline was developed by the National Collaborating Centre for Mental Health (NCCMH), which is a partnership between the Royal College of Psychiatrists and the British Psychological Society. The NCCMH worked with a group of healthcare professionals (from psychiatry, clinical psychology, mental health nursing, midwifery, health visiting, social work and general practice), former patients and technical staff, who reviewed the evidence and drafted the recommendations. In Scotland, SIGN recommend the establishment of pathways for referral and management of women with, or at risk of, mental illness in pregnancy and the postnatal period (Scottish Intercollegiate Guidelines Network, 2012).

Conclusions

There is a clear need for training of all health professionals in the nature, detection and treatment of perinatal depression, in understanding the experiences of the women, and in the development of listening skills and willingness to elicit and discuss psychological issues. For those implementing a postnatal depression service, training should include the use of the EPDS and how to administer it sensitively. Training should also include awareness of the risk of suicide in depression and guidelines on how to handle a positive response to item 10 on the EPDS.

Dealing with emotional problems can be taxing and training should be followed by ongoing support and consultation from a professional with counselling or therapy training. A range of prevention and intervention strategies should be explored, including individual and peer support, one-to-one counselling, antidepressants and the setting up of therapy or support groups in conjunction with mental healthcare staff.

CHAPTER 7

Using the Edinburgh Postnatal Depression Scale

This chapter summarises practical information for administering the EPDS based on research experience and on feedback from health professionals.

How to use the EPDS

1   Ask the woman to underline the response that comes closest to how she has felt during the previous 7 days.
2   Ensure that all ten items are completed.
3   The woman should complete the EPDS herself, unless she has difficulty with reading, and she should not discuss her answers with anyone other than the health professional when completing the scale.
4   The EPDS can be used routinely to screen for postnatal depression or to provide further information before referral of a woman who seems to have depression.
5   EPDS items are scored from 0 to 3; the normal response scores 0 and the 'severe' response scores 3. Total the individual item scores (see the EPDS scoring sheet in Appendix 1). Take care when scoring items and adding up the total as a recent study found between 13.4 and 28.9% of completed scales had errors (Matthey *et al*, 2013*b*).
6   A total score of 12 or above was taken in the three-centre study (Gerrard *et al*, 1994) as an indicator that the woman should be further assessed. Some authorities prefer a lower cut-off to ensure that depression is not missed (see Chapter 2).
7   Scores alone should not replace clinical judgement: women should be further assessed before deciding on treatment.

Using the EPDS in clinical practice

Routine use of the EPDS has a number of advantages.

1   It raises awareness of the possibility of postnatal depression among health professionals, women themselves and their families.

2   It may provide additional information when referring a woman to the GP or to the perinatal mental health team.

3   It can provide the opportunity for early preventive intervention.

4   It gives women 'permission to speak' and health professionals 'permission to listen'.

5   It can help a woman to recognise and discuss her negative feelings.

6   It may change women's perception of what health professionals can offer.

7   It can provide a structured approach to identification of low mood or depression, clarifying the situation for both the woman and the professional.

8   It can be used to monitor progress in treatment, and Matthey (2004) has calculated that a four-point reduction in the EPDS score is a clinically significant change.

9   It may help to prevent suicide.

10   It can lead to improved liaison with other professionals.

11   Evidence of the number of high-scoring women may alert health authorities and management to the need for extra services or redeployment of existing services.

The EPDS does not provide a differential diagnosis of mental disorder, neither can it replace clinical judgement. A high score does not necessarily imply that a woman has depression: she may simply be having a 'bad day', for example because of sleeplessness or temporary emotional or task overload. The opportunity to talk about her problems at a single interview may be sufficient to help her. Similarly, a low score does not always mean that a woman does not have depression: she may be unwilling or afraid to reveal her true feelings. One high score may indicate only that the woman is feeling temporarily overwhelmed by her circumstances or that she is tired and miserable on a particular day. Two high scores separated by 2 weeks, plus an interview, will usually confirm clinical depression.

Honesty of women's responses

There is no mystery about the meaning of the EPDS items, and it would certainly not be difficult to obtain a deliberately high or low score. In fact, the highest-scoring woman in our counselling trial (Holden *et al*, 1989) was assessed by the research psychiatrist as having a personality disorder: she enjoyed being the focus of attention. Health professionals have expressed particular concern about a total score of zero, especially if it seems that the woman is having problems: one would be very unlikely to obtain a zero score by answering honestly. However, as we have seen, the results of the EPDS validation studies (where an unseen EPDS score is compared with a diagnostic interview) indicate that most completed EPDS forms do accurately reflect the woman's feelings. If you are genuinely concerned, discuss the case with your line manager or the woman's family doctor.

What if someone does not wish to complete an EPDS?

There are many reasons why a woman may not wish to participate in screening. She may already be receiving treatment for depression; she may currently have depression but afraid to reveal her feelings in case of possible repercussions (a health professional's concern for the infant, referral, fear of stigmatisation); or she may not have depression and simply wishes to retain her privacy. Completing an EPDS is not compulsory. However, it does provide health professionals with an opportunity to identify women who may need help. The way the scale is presented is important, as is how the woman perceives that the information she reveals will be used. If a woman does not wish to avail herself of this opportunity, that is her absolute right and her wishes must be respected.

When, where and how should the EPDS be given?

Our original thinking (Cox *et al*, 1987) was that the EPDS could be given by health visitors during the postnatal check up in the GP's surgery or baby clinic at about 6 weeks, and this was done in our own research. In practice, we found that the 6-week EPDS picked up large numbers of women who, when interviewed by the research psychiatrist 4–6 weeks later, did not have depression. Although it has been shown (e.g. Seeley *et al*, 1996; Cooper & Murray, 1997) that early interventions lead to improved outcome for both mothers and their infants, at 6 weeks postnatally many women are still adjusting to the birth, to sleeplessness and to the turmoil of having a new infant. A large number of high scores are likely to be obtained if the EPDS is given routinely in the very early weeks, which may lead to intervention overload for health professionals.

Scottish Intercollegiate Guidelines Network

In their 2012 document on the management of perinatal mood disorders, SIGN recommends the guidelines issued by NICE for the detection of perinatal depression. SIGN's guidelines on when enquiry around depressive symptoms should be made are as follows:

- Enquiry about depressive symptoms should be made, at minimum, on booking in and postnatally at 4–6 weeks and 3–4 months.
- For women regarded to be at high risk (those with previous or current depressive disorder), enquiry about depressive symptoms should be made at each contact.
- The EPDS or the Whooley questions (see Chapter 6) may be used in the antenatal and postnatal period as an aid to clinical monitoring and to facilitate discussion of emotional issues.
- Where there are concerns about the presence of depression, women should be re-evaluated after 2 weeks. If symptoms persist, or if at

initial evaluation there is evidence of severe illness or suicidality, women should be referred to their GP or mental health service for further evaluation.

The CPHVA made the following recommendations for the use of the EPDS (Community Practitioners' and Health Visitors' Association, 2003):

1   The EPDS should never be used in isolation – it should form part of a full and systematic mood assessment of the mother, supporting professional judgement and a clinical interview.
2   The EPDS should be only used by professionals who have been trained in the detection and management of postnatal depression, use of the EPDS and conducting a clinical interview.
3   Formal mood assessments should only be carried out in a place where the mother is ensured privacy and when the professional has time to discuss the outcome and suitable interventions with the mother should they be necessary.
4   The EPDS should never be used in an open clinic or posted to mothers. If the clinic is not busy and there are facilities to ensure privacy for the mother it may be the preferred option for some health visitors unable to do a home visit.
5   Before using it the professional should consider possible factors which could influence the mother's comprehension of the purpose of the EPDS and her ability to complete the questions accurately, for example, literacy level, cultural background or language difficulties.
6   Having asked the mother to complete the scale, the professional should discuss the mother's individual responses one by one, being alert to a mismatch with her (or his) clinical impression, for example, mothers with puerperal psychosis may score low on the EPDS.
7   Use of the EPDS should be followed by a clinical interview that utilises the nine symptoms from DSM-IV to ascertain depressive symptoms. Such an interview should also explore physical, emotional or social causes for the symptoms so that appropriate interventions can be discussed with the mother.

A specific score on the EPDS does not definitely confirm or refute the presence of postnatal depression. What it does offer is an indicator as to its possible presence, absence or severity. Is it reasonable, then, to consider whether much attention should be given to the score? The CPHVA believes that the score does have a quantitative value to the service provider, as when it is recorded it can support a needs assessment for service provision. It also serves as a benchmark for changes in the mother's mood or in response to a change in service. We believe that from the individual mother's viewpoint, while noting the score, the health visitor should rely on her fuller mood assessment to determine the severity of any depression.

We regard this important policy statement by the CPHVA as consistent with the recommendations in this book. The debate initiated by the National Screening Committee is a potent spur to further develop the evidence base for a perinatal mental health service.

Taking action on high scores

Any woman who scores above the chosen threshold should be given the opportunity for further discussion and assessment, usually within 2 weeks (follow local policy guidelines). Encourage her to talk about her responses to the EPDS items and about her feelings generally. If, on assessment, it seems clear that her low mood is temporary, reassure her that you and her family doctor are available for further help and let her know how to contact you if she feels the need.

A repeated high score 2 weeks later almost certainly indicates depression and the need for further assessment and intervention. A woman who has more than a transient low mood should be persuaded to see her doctor for assessment. A set number of extra weekly supportive listening visits may be offered by the health visitor and/or antidepressants may be prescribed by the family doctor. The woman should be reviewed using the EPDS after an appropriate time interval. Women who do not respond to these simple measures may need to see a psychologist or be referred for further psychiatric assessment.

See Chapter 6 for a discussion on what to do if an individual has any score on item 10, which indicates suicidal feelings.

Electronic EPDS

Computerised versions of the EPDS were first produced and validated by Glaze & Cox (1991). They reported that women were quite happy to complete the scale in this way. Computerisation reduces demand on staff time and permits introduction of the EPDS even when staffing levels are low. Among the disadvantages of the computerised EPDS are that staff might require training in the use of the computer, that data protection needs special attention and that, unless laptops are provided, administration would be restricted to one setting (so that mothers with depression, who are often unwilling to leave their homes, would be missed (Elliott, 1994)). Since then, an internet version has been validated (Spek *et al*, 2008), and with the advent of smart phones and tablet computers, taking the electronic version to the woman has become easier. A small mixed-methods study has explored the use of an online version of the EPDS: after receiving an email prompt, the woman completes it and then receives the score and referral information (Drake *et al*, 2013). The authors suggest this can reduce the stigma associated with depression as it can be done privately, and also improves access for rural and disadvantaged women.

Antenatal use

The EPDS may also be used in pregnancy, either routinely or to identify suspected depression. In our three-centre training study (Gerrard *et al*, 1994), we asked health visitors to give an EPDS to every woman at about 28 weeks antenatally, both to introduce the idea that health professionals are concerned with women's emotional well-being and to detect depression. In Murray & Cox's (1990) validation of the EPDS in pregnancy, midwives screened all pregnant women, as they did in the Cambridge prenatal study (Green, 1998) and in the Avon study reported by Evans *et al* (2001). As Evans *et al* point out, however, the benefits of routine antenatal screening have not yet been demonstrated by research.

Who should give the EPDS?

Although our research in the UK has concentrated on the use of the EPDS by health visitors and midwives, it can be administered by any health professional who understands its use, including doctors, psychologists, midwives and community psychiatric nurses. Irrespective of who administers the scale, the importance of a team approach to intervention cannot be overemphasised.

Record-keeping

Where to keep completed EPDS forms should be a management decision, but as a general rule, information about the mother should always be kept with her own health records, not with those of the infant. Remember that this material is strictly confidential. It should not be divulged to anyone outside the healthcare team without the woman's knowledge and consent.

Using the EPDS with non-English speakers

A translation of the EPDS or the English-language version explained by an interpreter may be used to open the subject for discussion, but only a validated translation may be assumed to give scores that have the same meaning as those from the original English. Cultural differences in interpretation might result in a score that does not accurately reflect the mother's mood (see Chapter 3).

Using the EPDS in research

The EPDS continues to be used extensively in research. Research uses include: determining the percentage of women with low mood, investigating the correlates of low mood and determining risk factors; first-stage screening in epidemiological community studies; identifying women with depression for an intervention trial; monitoring changes over time in depressive symptoms in clinical intervention trials; and/or determining the need for intervention.

Some studies report that 'depression was measured using the EPDS'. This is incorrect: a single EPDS score above threshold does not indicate that a woman has depression, only that sufficient depressive symptoms are present to make this likely. If the EPDS is used as a stand-alone measure, then it can be claimed only that women did or did not have scores above the chosen threshold. For some studies this is acceptable. However, in studies in which it is important to know whether women currently have depression (such as recruitment to an intervention trial, or measuring the success or otherwise of an intervention), the scale should be accompanied by a reliable clinical assessment interview.

Misuse of the EPDS

Variations in the cut-off used, the title, wording and format of the scale, and omitting some of the ten items have all been reported (Matthey *et al*, 2006). Not all these changes have been validated, so the impact may be unknown. One change in format (using tick boxes instead of underlining the correct answer) led to women in a qualitative study reporting finding the version used (six items in a three-by-two format with tick boxes and with no explanatory introductory paragraph) 'impersonal', 'crude', 'brutal', 'blunt' and 'clumsy' (Cubison & Munro, 2005). It must be stressed that to call any variant of the original scale the EPDS is a breach of copyright and the original 10-item scale should only be referred to as 'The Edinburgh Postnatal Depression Scale'.

Conclusions

It must be emphasised that the EPDS is only a screen for depression. It reveals low mood at the time of completion and indicates a need for further assessment. It does not provide a differential diagnosis of mental disorder and does not replace clinical judgement. Screening does not in itself constitute an intervention, nor, on its own, does it improve outcomes; it does give an indication of a woman's need for help and should be a precursor to diagnosis and intervention. Adequate training, support and cooperation between service providers are needed to develop a structured and effective approach to promoting the psychological well-being of women during the postnatal period.

Routine use of the EPDS in healthcare settings may prevent much suffering by identifying women who need treatment and reassuring those whose low mood is temporary. It might also help to persuade women that it is safe to talk about negative feelings.

The Edinburgh Postnatal Depression Scale

How are you feeling?

As you have recently had a baby, we would like to know how you are feeling now. Please <u>underline</u> the answer which comes closest to how you have felt in the past 7 days, not just how you feel today. Here is an example, already completed:

I have felt happy:
Yes, most of the time
<u>Yes, some of the time</u>
No, not very often
No, not at all

This would mean: 'I have felt happy some of the time during the past week'. Please complete the other questions in the same way.

In the past 7 days

1. I have been able to laugh and see the funny side of things:
   As much as I always could
   Not quite so much now
   Definitely not so much now
   Not at all

2. I have looked forward with enjoyment to things:
   As much as I ever did
   Rather less than I used to
   Definitely less than I used to
   Hardly at all

3. I have blamed myself unnecessarily when things went wrong:
    Yes, most of the time
    Yes, some of the time
    Not very often
    No, never

4. I have been anxious or worried for no good reason:
    No, not at all
    Hardly ever
    Yes, sometimes
    Yes, very often

5. I have felt scared or panicky for no very good reason:
    Yes, quite a lot
    Yes, sometimes
    No, not much
    No, not at all

6. Things have been getting on top of me:
    Yes, most of the time I haven't been able to cope at all
    Yes, sometimes I haven't been coping as well as usual
    No, most of the time I have coped quite well
    No, I have been coping as well as ever

7. I have been so unhappy that I have had difficulty sleeping:
    Yes, most of the time
    Yes, sometimes
    Not very often
    No, not at all

8. I have felt sad or miserable:
    Yes, most of the time
    Yes, quite often
    Not very often
    No, not at all

9. I have been so unhappy that I have been crying:
    Yes, most of the time
    Yes, quite often
    Only occasionally
    No, never

10. The thought of harming myself has occurred to me:
    Yes, quite often
    Sometimes
    Hardly ever
    Never

Edinburgh Postnatal Depression Scale: scoring sheet

1. I have been able to laugh and see the funny side of things:
As much as I always could	0
Not quite so much now	1
Definitely not so much now	2
Not at all	3

2. I have looked forward with enjoyment to things:
As much as I ever did	0
Rather less than I used to	1
Definitely less than I used to	2
Hardly at all	3

3. I have blamed myself unnecessarily when things went wrong:
Yes, most of the time	3
Yes, some of the time	2
Not very often	1
No, never	0

4. I have been anxious or worried for no good reason:
No, not at all	0
Hardly ever	1
Yes, sometimes	2
Yes, very often	3

5. I have felt scared or panicky for no very good reason:
Yes, quite a lot	3
Yes, sometimes	2
No, not much	1
No, not at all	0

6. Things have been getting on top of me:
Yes, most of the time I haven't been able to cope at all	3
Yes, sometimes I haven't been coping as well as usual	2
No, most of the time I have coped quite well	1
No, I have been coping as well as ever	0

7. I have been so unhappy that I have had difficulty sleeping:
Yes, most of the time	3
Yes, sometimes	2
Not very often	1
No, not at all	0

8. I have felt sad or miserable:
Yes, most of the time	3
Yes, quite often	2
Not very often	1
No, not at all	0

9. I have been so unhappy that I have been crying:

    Yes, most of the time   3

    Yes, quite often   2

    Only occasionally   1

    No, never   0

10. The thought of harming myself has occurred to me:

    Yes, quite often   3

    Sometimes   2

    Hardly ever   1

    Never   0

Translations of the Edinburgh Postnatal Depression Scale

The English-language Edinburgh Postnatal Depression Scale (EPDS) has been widely translated and this appendix reproduces some of these translations. Key references, including validation studies where applicable, are given for each translation. A full list of all the translations we are aware of is given in Chapter 3. The authors and publishers cannot vouch for the validity of any translations that have not undergone a positive validation, and would be grateful for any additional information on validation studies using these translations. Please contact the publishers if you wish to translate the EPDS into any language not listed below.

- Afaan Oromo (source unknown)
- Amharic (Hanlon et al, 2008)
- Arabic (United Arab Emirates: Ghubash *et al*, 1997; Morocco: Agoub *et al*, 2005)
- Bangla (Gausia *et al*, 2007)
- Chichewa (Stewart *et al*, 2013)
- Chinese (Hong Kong: Lee *et al*, 1998; Taiwan: Heh, 2001; Teng *et al*, 2005; mainland China: Wang *et al*, 2009; Lau *et al*, 2010)
- Czech (Dragonas *et al*, 1996)
- Dari (Shafiei *et al*, 2011)
- Dutch (Pop *et al*, 1992)
- Estonian (source unknown)
- Farsi/Persian (Montazeri *et al*, 2007; Kheirabadi *et al*, 2012)
- Filipino/Tagalog (Small *et al*, 2003)
- Finnish (source unknown)

- French (Guedeney & Fermanian, 1998; Quebec, Canada: Des Rivières-Pigeon *et al*, 2000)
- German (Austria: Herz *et al*, 1997; Bergant *et al*, 1998; Muzik *et al*, 2000)
- Greek (Thorpe *et al*, 1992; Leonardou *et al*, 2009; Vivilaki *et al*, 2009)
- Hebrew (Katzenelson *et al*, 2000)
- Hindi (Banerjee *et al*, 2000)
- Hungarian (Töreki *et al*, 2013)
- Icelandic (Thome, 1992, 1996, 1999)
- Igbo (Uwakwe & Okonkwo, 2003)
- Indonesian (source unknown)
- Italian (Carpiniello *et al*, 1997; Benvenuti *et al*, 1999)
- Japanese (Okano *et al*, 1996, 1998, 2005; Yoshida *et al*, 2001)
- Kannada (Fernandes *et al*, 2011)
- Khmer/Cambodia (Fitzgerald *et al*, 1998)
- Konkani (Patel *et al*, 2003)
- Korean (Kim & Buist, 2005)
- Kurdish (Ahmed *et al*, 2012)
- Lithuanian (Bunevicius *et al*, 2009)
- Macedonian (source unknown)
- Malay (Rushidi *et al*, 2002; Mahmud *et al*, 2003; Kadir *et al*, 2004)
- Maltese (Felice *et al*, 2006)
- Myanmar/Burmese (source unknown)
- Nepali (Regmi *et al*, 2002)
- Norwegian (Eberhard-Gran *et al*, 2001; Berle *et al*, 2003)
- Polish (Bielawska-Batorowicz, 1995)
- Portuguese (Portugal: Areias *et al*, 1996*a*; Brazil: Da-Silva *et al*, 1998; Santos *et al*, 2007*b*)
- Punjabi (Clifford *et al*, 1997, 1999; Werrett & Clifford, 2006)
- Romanian (Wallis *et al*, 2012)
- Russian (Glasser *et al*, 1998)
- Samoan (Ekeroma *et al*, 2012)
- Serbian (source unknown)
- Slovenian (M. Blinc Pesek, personal communication, 2003)
- Somali (source unknown)
- Spanish (Chile: Jadresic *et al*, 1995; Peru: Vega-Dienstmaier *et al*, 2002; Spain: Ascaso Terrén *et al*, 2003; Garcia-Esteve *et al*, 2003; Mexico: Alvarado-Esquivel *et al*, 2006)
- Swedish (Lundh & Gyllang, 1993; Wickberg & Hwang, 1996*a*)
- Tamil (Benjamin *et al*, 2005)
- Thai (Pitanupong *et al*, 2007)
- Turkish (Aydin *et al*, 2004)
- Twi (Weobong *et al*, 2009)
- Urdu (Bannerjee *et al*, 2000)
- Vietnamese (Matthey *et al*, 1997; Tran *et al*, 2011)
- Xhosa (de Bruin *et al*, 2004)

Afaan Oromo – Ethiopia

Maaltuu sitti dhaga'amaa jira?

Dhiheenya kana mucaa da'uu kee irraa kan ka'e amma maaltuu akka sitti dhaga'amaa jiru baruu barbaanna. Maaloo kan har'a sitti dhaga'ame qofa osoo hintaane, guyyaa 7 darban keessa kan sitti dhaga'amaa ture deebii ibsuu danda'u yokaan ammoo kan itti dhihaatu jala muti. Fakeenyi armaan gadii akkaata deebichi itti guutamu agarsiisa.

> Ani gammadaan jira:
> > Eyyee, yeroo hedduu nan gammada
> > Eyyee, yeroo tokko-tokko nan gammada
> > Lakkii, yeroo hedduu miti hingammadu
> > Lakkii, yeroo tokkoyyuu hingammadu.

Kana jechuun: 'torban darbe keessa yeroo tokko tokko gammadaan turee jechuudha'.

Maaloo gaaffilee kaanis akkataadhuma fakkeenya kanaan guuti.

Guyyaa 7 darbaan keessatti

1. Kolfuu fi waan nama kofalchiisan arguu danda'eera:
    Hanguman yeroo kaan godhuu danda'u
    Hanga yeroo kaanii gochuu hindanda'u
    Amma yeroo hedduu hinkolfu
    Amma tasumaa hinkolfu

2. Gammachuudhanin waan tokko-tokko gara fuul-duraatti ilaalaa jira:
    Hangumaan duraan godhaa ture
    Kanaan duraan godhu irraa gadi
    Kan duraanii irraa haalan gadi
    Tasuma akkas hingodhu

3. Yeroo waan tokko tokko karaa irraa ka'atan gar-maleen of balaaleffadha:
    Eyyee, yeroo hedduu
    Eyyee, yeroo tokko-tokko
    Lakkii, yeroo hedduu miti
    Lakkii, tasumaa akkana hingodhu

4. Sababa gahoo/amansiisoo hintaaneefin yeroo hedduu cinqama:
    Lakkii, tasayyuu akkana hingodhu
    Hedduu akkas godhee hinbeeku
    Eyyee, yeroo tokko-tokko
    Eyyee, yeroo hedduu

© The Royal College of Psychiatrists 1987. Translated from Cox JL, Holden JM, Sagovsky R (1987) Detection of postnatal depression. Development of the 10-item Edinburgh Postnatal Depression Scale. *British Journal of Psychiatry*, **150**, 782–786.

5. Sodaanii fi naasuun sababa gahoo/amansiisoo malee natti dhaga'amu:
   Eyyee, yeroo hedduu
   Eyyee, yeroo tokko-tokko
   Lakkii, yeroo hedduu miti
   Lakkii, tasayyuu natti hindhaga'aman

6. Waanni marti na yaaddeesu:
   Eyyee, yerooo hedduu irraa dandamachuu hindandeenye
   Eyyee, yeroo tokko-tokko akka duri kiyyaatti irraa dandamachuu hindandeenye
   Lakkii, yeroo hedduu akkuma duraanii kiyyaatti garrii godheen dandamamachaa jira
   Lakiii, akkuma duraanii kiyyaatti garii godhee dandamachaan jira

7. Gar-malee gammachuu qabaachaa waanan hinjirreef irriba rafuu irratti rakkina qabaachaan jira:
   Eyyee, yeroo hedduu
   Eyyee, irra deddeebi'ee
   Yeroo hedduu miti
   Lakkii, tasa akkasi ta'ee hinbeeku

8. Gaddi yokaan ammoo yaadni samuu nama rakku natti dhaga'amaa jira:
   Eyyee, yeroo hedduu
   Eyyee, irra deddeebi'ee
   Yeroo hedduu miti
   Lakkii, tasa akkas godhee hinbeeku

9. Waanaan gammachuu qabaachaa hinjirreef na boosisaa jira:
   Eyyee, yeroo hedduu
   Eyyee, irra deddeebi'ee
   Yeroo tokko-tokkko qofa
   Lakki, tasa akkas godhee hinbeeku

10. Yaadni 'ofi-miidhi' naan jedhu natti dhaga'amaa jira
    Eyyee, irra deddeebi'ee
    Yeroo tokko-tokko
    Hedduu miti
    Ta'ee hinbeeku

Amharic

1) ባለፈው ሳምንት ውስጥ የነገሮችን አስቂኝ ሁኔታ በማየት ለመሣቅ ችለው ነበር?

አዎን: [ ] መልሳቸው አዎን ከሆነ (ጠይቅ)	ሁልጊዜ የማደርገውን ያህል? [ ] 0
የለም: [ ] መልሳቸው የለም ከሆነ (ጠይቅ)	ባሁኑ ጊዜ የድርውን ያህል አልችልም [ ] 1 በርግጠኝነት የድርውን ያህል አልችልም ነበር [ ] 2 ፍጹም አልችልም ነበር [ ] 3

2) ባለፈው ሳምንት ውስጥ ነገሮችን በደስታ /በናፍቆት /ሲጠባበቁ ነበር?

አዎን: [ ] መልሳቸው አዎን ከሆነ (ጠይቅ)	ከዚህ በፊት እንደማደርገው ያህል [ ] 0
የለም: [ ] መልሳቸው የለም ከሆነ (ጠይቅ)	በመጠኑ በፊት ከማደርገው በቀነሰ ሁኔታ [ ] 1 በርግጠኝነት በፊት ከማደርገው ባነሰ መጠን [ ] 2 በፍጹም አልጠባበትም ነበር [ ] 3

3) ባለፈው ሳምንት ውስጥ አንዳንድ ነገሮች ሣይሳኩ ሲቀር ያለአግባብ ራስዎን ይወቅሱ ነበር?

አዎን: [ ] መልሳቸው አዎን ከሆነ (ጠይቅ)	አዎን አብዛኛው ጊዜ [ ] 3 አዎን አንዳንድ ጊዜ [ ] 2 በጣም ጥቂት ጊዜ [ ] 1
የለም: [ ] መልሳቸው የለም ከሆነ (ጠይቅ)	አይ በፍጹም አልነበረም [ ] 0

4) ባለፈው ሳምንት ውስጥ ያለ በቂ ምክንያት ሲጨነቁ ወይም ሲሰጉ ነበር?

አዎን: [ ] መልሳቸው አዎን ከሆነ (ጠይቅ)	አም አብዛኛውን ጊዜ [ ] 0 አም አንዳንዴ [ ] 1
የለም: [ ] መልሳቸው የለም ከሆነ (ጠይቅ)	በእምብዛም አያጋጥመኝም [ ] 2 አይ አጋጥሞኝ አያውቅም [ ] 3

5) ባለፈው ሳምንት ውስጥ ያለ በቂ ምክንያት የመፍራት: የመሸበር: ድንጋጥ ድንግጥ የማለት ስሜት ይሰማዎት ነበር?

አዎን: [ ] መልሳቸው አዎን ከሆነ (ጠይቅ)	አም ብዙውን ጊዜ [ ] 3 አዎን አንዳንድ ጊዜ [ ] 2 በጣም ጥቂት ጊዜ [ ] 1
የለም: [ ] መልሳቸው የለም ከሆነ (ጠይቅ)	አይ ፍጹም አልነበረም [ ] 0

6) ባለፈው ሳምንት ውስጥ ነገሮች ሁሉ ከአቅምም በላይ እየሆኑብዎ ነበር?

አዎን: [ ] መልሳቸው አዎን ከሆነ (ጠይቅ)	አም ብዙ ጊዜ መቋቋም አልቻልኩም [ ] 3 አም አንድ አንድ ጊዜ መቋቋም አልቻልኩም [ ] 2
የለም: [ ] መልሳቸው የለም ከሆነ (ጠይቅ)	የለም ብዙ ጊዜ መቋቋም ችያለሁ [ ] 1 የለም እንደወትሮዬ መቋቋም ችያለሁ [ ] 0

7) ባለፈው ሳምንት ውስጥ ደስታ በማጣ ከማጣት የተነሳ የእንቅልፍ ችግር ነበረብዎ?

አዎን: [ ] መልሳቸው አዎን ከሆነ (ጠይቅ)	አዎን አብዛኛው ጊዜ [ ] 3 አዎን አነዳንድ ጊዜ [ ] 2
የለም: [ ] መልሳቸው የለም ከሆነ (ጠይቅ)	የለም በጣም ጥቂት ጊዜ [ ] 1 የለም ፈጽሞ አልነበረም [ ] 0

8) ባለፈው ሳምንት ውስጥ የመከፋት ወይም የመሪር ሀዘን ስሜት ይሰማዎ ነበር?

አዎን: [ ] መልሳቸው አዎን ከሆነ (ጠይቅ)	አዎን በአብዛኛውን ጊዜ [ ] 3 አዎን በመጠኑ ብዙ ጊዜ [ ] 2
የለም: [ ] መልሳቸው የለም ከሆነ (ጠይቅ)	የለም በጣም ብዙ ጊዜ አልነበረም [ ] 1 የለም ፈጽሞ አልነበረም [ ] 0

9) ባለፈው ሳምንት ውስጥ ደስታ በማጣ ከማጣት የተነሣ አልቅሰው ነበር?

አዎን: [ ] መልሳቸው አዎን ከሆነ (ጠይቅ)	አዎን በአብዛኛውን ጊዜ [ ] 3 አዎን በመጠኑ ብዙ ጊዜ [ ] 2 አልፎ አልፎ ብቻ [ ] 1
የለም: [ ] መልሳቸው የለም ከሆነ (ጠይቅ)	የለም ፈጽሞ አልነበረም [ ] 0

10) ባለፈው ሳምንት ውስጥ በሕይወትም ላይ ጉዳት ለማድረስ አስበው ነበር?

አዎን: [ ] መልሳቸው አዎን ከሆነ (ጠይቅ)	አዎን ብዙ ጊዜ [ ] 3 አንዳንድ ጊዜ [ ] 2
የለም: [ ] መልሳቸው የለም ከሆነ (ጠይቅ)	እምብዛም አስቤ አላውቅም [ ] 1 በፍጹም አላሰብኩም [ ] 0

Arabic

سيدتي
الرجاء أن تضعي خطا تحت الجواب الذي يعبر بطريقة أدق عن كيفية شعورك في الأيام السبعة الماضية، وليس عن شعورك اليوم فحسب.

إليك مثل وقد أكمل:

لقد شعرت بأنني سعيدة
ـ نعم كل الأوقات
ـ نعم معظم الأوقات
ـ كلا ليس في أحوال كثيرة
ـ كلا أبدا

وهذا يعني : لقد شعرت بأنني سعيدة معظم الوقت خلال الأسبوع الماضي. الرجاء أن تكملي الأسئلة الأخرى بالطريقة ذاتها.

نرجو أن تضعي خطا تحت أحد الأجوبة التالية:
خلال الأيام السبعة الماضية

1. لقد استطعت الشعور بالفرح والسعادة
ـ بالمقدار نفسه الذي استطعته قبلا
ـ ليس تماما بالمقدار نفسه الآن
ـ قطعا ليس بالمقدار نفسه الآن
ـ كلا مطلقا

2. لقد تطلعت الى الأمور بتمتع
ـ بالمقدار نفسه مثل أي وقت مضى
ـ أقل نوعا ما مما اعتدته
ـ قطعا أقل مما اعتدته
ـ نادرا. أبدا

3. لقد لمت نفسي بدون لزوم عندما سارت الأمور على غير ما يرام
ـ نعم في معظم الأحيان
ـ نعم في بعض الأحيان
ـ ليس في أحوال كثيرة
ـ كلا أبدا

4. لقد كنت قلقة ومشغولة البال بدون سبب وجيه
- كلا أبدا
- نادرا
- نعم في بعض الأحيان
- نعم في احوال كثيرة

5. لقد شعرت بالخوف والذعر بدون سبب وجيه
- نعم أكثر الأحيان
- نعم في بعض الأحيان
- كلا ليس كثيرا
- كلا مطلقا

6. تراكمت الأعمال علي فلم أستطع القيام بها كلها
- نعم في معظم الأحيان لم أستطع أبدا القيام بها
- نعم في بعض الأحيان لم أستطع القيام بها كالمعتاد
- كلا لقد استطعت القيام بها في بعض الأحيان
- كلا لقد استطعت القيام بها كالمعتاد

7. لقد كنت غير سعيدة لدرجة أنه كانت لدي صعوبة في النوم
- نعم في معظم الأحيان
- نعم في بعض الأحيان
- ليس كثيرا
- كلا أبدا

8. لقد شعرت بأنني لست سعيدة وبائسة
- نعم في معظم الأحيان
- نعم أكثر الأحيان
- كلا ليس أكثر الأحيان
- كلا مطلقا

9. لقد كنت غير سعيدة وأشعر بألم مرير لدرجة كنت ابكي
- نعم في معظم الأحيان
- نعم أكثر الأحيان
- فقط من وقت الى آخر
- كلا أبدا

10. لقد خطرت لي فكرة الحاق الأذى بنفسي
- نعم في احوال كثيرة
- نعم في بعض الأحيان
- نادرا
- كلا مطلقا

Bangla

সম্প্রতি আপনার একটি বাচ্চা হয়েছে, আমরা জানতে চাচ্ছি আপনার কেমন লাগছে। শুধু আজকে আপনার কেমন লাগছে তা নয় বরং **গত এক সপ্তাহ (৭ দিন) ধরে** আপনার কেমন অনুভব হচ্ছে তা কি দয়া করে আমাদেরকে বলবেন। এজন্য আমরা আপনাকে ১০টি প্রশ্ন করবো। প্রতিটি প্রশ্নের ৪টি করে উত্তর থাকবে, যে উত্তরটা আপনার সঙ্গে মিলে যাবে বা কাছাকাছি হবে সেটাই বলুন।

একটি উদাহরন দিচ্ছি - আপনি আনন্দে ছিলেন:

- ০ হ্যা, সব সময়ই
- ● হ্যা, বেশীরভাগ সময়ই
- ০ না,প্রায়ই না
- ০ না, একেবারেই না

(●) এটার অর্থ হচ্ছে "আপনি গত সপ্তায় বেশীরভাগ সময় আনন্দে ছিলেন"

এভাবে নিম্নলিখিত প্রশ্নগুলোর উত্তর দিন:

১. আপনি হাসতে পেরেছেন এবং হাসি - তামাসা উপভোগ করতে পেরেছেন

- ০ যতটুকু আপনি সব সময় করেছেন
- ০ এখন আগের মত ততটা না
- ০ অবশ্যই এখন ততটা না
- ০ একেবারেই না

২. আপনি সবকিছু থেকে আন ন্দ পাওয়ার আশায় থেকেছেন

- ০ যতটুকু আপনি আগে করতেন
- ০ আগের চেয়ে কিছু কম
- ০ অবশ্যই আগের চেয়ে কম
- ০ বলতে গেলে একেবারেই না

৩. কোন কিছু ঠিকমত না হলে আপনি নিজেকে অ-যথাই দোষ দিয়ে থাকেন

- ০ হ্যা, বেশিরভাগ সময়
- ০ হ্যা, মাঝে মাঝে
- ০ খুব বেশি না
- ০ না,কখনোই না

৪. আপনি অকারনে দুশ্চিন্তা করে থাকেন বা ঘাবড়িয়ে যান

- ০ না, কখনোই না
- ০ খুবই কম
- ০ হ্যা, মাঝে মাঝে
- ০ হ্যা, প্রায়ই

৫. আপনি অকারনে ভয় পেয়েছেন ও আতঙ্কিত হয়েছেন

      ○ হ্যা, খুব বেশি
      ○ হ্যা, মাঝে মাঝে
      ○ না, বেশি না
      ○ না, একেবারেই না

৬. সবকিছু আপনার কাছে বোঝা মনে হয়েছে

      ○ হ্যা, বেশিরভাগ সময়ই আপনি মানিয়ে নিতে পারছেন না
      ○ হ্যা, মাঝে মাঝে আপনি মানিয়ে নিতে পারছেন না, যেমন আপনি
          সাধারনতঃ নিয়ে থাকেন
      ○ না, বেশিরভাগ সময়ই আপনি ভালভাবে মানিয়ে নিচ্ছেন
      ○ না, আপনি সব সময় ভালভাবেই মানিয়ে নিচ্ছেন

৭. আপনার মনটা এতোই খারাপ ছিল যে, আপনার ঘুমের অসুবিধা হয়েছে

      ○ হ্যা, বেশিরভাগ সময়ই
      ○ হ্যা, মাঝে মাঝে
      ○ প্রায়ই না
      ○ না , একেবারেই না

৮. আপনার নিজেকে দুঃখী বা অসহায় মনে হয়েছে

      ○ হ্যা, বেশিরভাগ সময়ই
      ○ হ্যা, প্রায় প্রায়ই
      ○ না,প্রায়ই না
      ○ না, একেবারেই না

৯. আপনার মনটা এতোই খারাপ ছিল যে আপনি কেঁদেছেন

      ○ হ্যা, বেশিরভাগ সময়ই
      ○ হ্যা, প্রায় প্রায়ই
      ○ কখনো কখনো
      ○ না, কখনোই না

১০. আপনি নিজেই নিজের ক্ষতি করার কথা ভেবেছেন

      ○ হ্যা,প্রায়ই
      ○ মাঝে মাঝে
      ○ খুবই কম
      ○ কখনোই না

Chichewa

Tsopano ndikufunsani mafunso am'mene mwakhala mukuganizila ndikumvera masiku asanu ndi awiri apitawa. Mafunso awiri oyambilira tigwilitsa ntchito mbali imodzi ya kadi. Chithunzi chilichonse chikuimila limodzi mwa mayankho anayi. Ndidziloza zithunzi ndikamawelenga mayankho a funso lililonse. Musankhe yankho logwilidzana ndi m'mene mwakhala mukumvela masiku asanu ndi awiri apitawa.

1. *Masiku asanu ndi awiri apitawa,* kodi mwakhala mukutha kuseka komanso kuona kusangalatsa kwa zinthu?
   - ☐ [1] Olo mpang'ono komwe
   - ☐ [2] Panopa osati kwambiri
   - ☐ [1] Osati bwino kwambiri
   - ☐ [0] Monga m'mene mumathera nthawi zonse

2. *Masiku asanu ndi awiri apitawa,* kodi mwakhala mukudikira ndi nsangala mu zinthu zozachitika mtsogolo?
   - ☐ [1] Olo mpang'ono komwe
   - ☐ [2] Panopa osati kwambiri
   - ☐ [1] Osati bwino kwambiri
   - ☐ [0] Monga m'mene mumathera nthawi zonse

Mafunso otsatilawa tigwilisa ntchito mbali yachiwiri ya kadi. Mobwelenzanso,chithunzi chilichonse chikuimila limodzi mwa mayankho anayi. Ndiziloza zithunzi ndikamawelenga mayankho a funso lililonse. Musankhe yankho logwilizana ndi m'mene mwakhala mukumvela masiku asanu ndi awiri apitawa

3. *Masiku asanu ndi awiri apitawa,* kodi mumazida nokha mosafunikila pamene zinthu sizinayendebwino?
   - ☐ [3] Nthawi zambiri
   - ☐ [2] Kawirikawiri
   - ☐ [1] Mwakamodzikamodzi
   - ☐ [0] Sizinachitikepo

4. *Masiku asanu ndi awiri apitawa,* kodi mumakhumudwa kapena kudela nkhawa popanda chifukwa chenicheni?
   - ☐ [3] Kwambiri
   - ☐ [2] Nthawi zina
   - ☐ [1] Sizimachitika
   - ☐ [0] Olo mpang'ono pomwe

5. *Masiku asanu ndi awiri apitawa,* kodi mumachita mantha kapena kusowa mtendere popanda chifukwa chenicheni?
   - ☐ [3] Kwambiri
   - ☐ [2] Nthawi zina
   - ☐ [1] Osati kwambiri
   - ☐ [0] Ngakhale pang'ono

6. *Masiku asanu ndi awiri apitawa,* kodi mwakhala mukuganiza kapena kumva ngati munalindi zinthu zambiri zoyenela kuchita koma simumakwanisa kuchita ?
   - ☐ [3] Nthawi zambiri mwakhala mukulepheratu
   - ☐ [2] Nthawi zina mwakhala mukulepheratu
   - ☐ [1] Nthawi zambiri mwakhala mukutha
   - ☐ [0] Mwakhala mukutha ngati m'mene mumapangira nthawi

7. *Masiku asanu ndi awiri apitawa,* kodi mwakhala osasangalala moti mwakhala mukulephera kugona?
   ☐ [3] Nthawi zambiri
   ☐ [2] Kawirikawiri
   ☐ [1] Osati kawirikawiri
   ☐ [0] Mpang'ono pomwe

8. *Masiku asanu ndi awiri apitawa,* kodi munali wokhumudwa kapena kusowa mtendere wa mumtima?
   ☐ [3] Nthawi zambiri
   ☐ [2] Kawirikawiri
   ☐ [1] Osati kawirikawiri
   ☐ [0] Mpang'ono pomwe

9. *Masiku asanu ndi awiri apitawa,* kodi mwakhala osasangalala moti mwakhala mukulira?
   ☐ [3] Nthawi zambiri
   ☐ [2] Kawirikawiri
   ☐ [1] Mwakamodzikamodzi
   ☐ [0] Sizinachitikepo

10. *Masiku asanu ndi awiri apitawa,* kodi munakhalapo ndi maganizo ofuna kuzipweteka?
    ☐ [3] Nthawi zambiri
    ☐ [2] Kawirikawiri
    ☐ [1] Mwakamodzikamodzi
    ☐ [0] Sizinachitikepo

[3]   [2]   [1]   [0]

EPDS: **QUESTIONS 1 AND 2** RESPONSE CARD

[3]   [2]   [1]   [0]

EPDS: **QUESTIONS 3 - 10** RESPONSE CARD

Chinese (Mandarin)

得分

愛丁堡產後抑鬱量表(HK-EPDS2.0a)

姓名 _____ 年齡 _____ 新生孩子周歲 _____ 填表日期

說明：因爲您剛生了孩子，我們想了解一下您的感受。請選擇一個最能反映您過去七天感受的答案。

注意：不只是您今天的感覺，而是過去七天的感受。例如：

我感到愉快。　　（1）所有時候這樣。

　　　　　　　　（2）大部分時候這樣。

　　　　　　　　（3）不經常這樣。

　　　　　　　　（4）一點也沒有。

選擇答案（2）表明在上一周內你大部分時間都感到愉快。請照同樣方法完成以下各題。

在過去七天內：

1. 我能看到事物有趣的一面，並笑得開心。
   - （1）　同以前一樣。
   - （2）　沒有以前那麼多。
   - （3）　肯定比以前少。
   - （4）　完全不能。

2. 我欣然期待未來的一切。
   - （1）　同以前一樣。
   - （2）　沒有以前那麼多。
   - （3）　肯定比以前少。
   - （4）　完全不能。

3. 當事情出錯時，我會不必要地責備自己。
   - （1）　大部分時候這樣。
   - （2）　有時候這樣。
   - （3）　不經常這樣。
   - （4）　沒有這樣。

4. 我無緣無故感到焦慮和擔心。
   - （1）　一點也沒有。
   - （2）　極少有。
   - （3）　有時候這樣。
   - （4）　經常這樣。

5. 我無緣無故感到害怕和驚慌。
   - （1）　相當多時候這樣。
   - （2）　有時候這樣。
   - （3）　不經常這樣。
   - （4）　一點也沒有。

6. 很多事情衝著我而來，使我透不過氣。
   - （1）　大多數時候我都不能應付。
   - （2）　有時候我不能像平時那樣應付得好。
   - （3）　大部分時候我都能像平時那樣應付得好。
   - （4）　我一直都能應付得好。

7. 我很不開心，以致失眠。
   - （1）　大部分時候這樣。
   - （2）　有時候這樣。
   - （3）　不經常這樣。
   - （4）　一點也沒有。

8. 我感到難過和悲傷。
   - （1）　大部分時候這樣。
   - （2）　相當時候這樣。
   - （3）　不經常這樣。
   - （4）　一點也沒有。

9. 我不開心到哭。
   - （1）　大部分時候這樣。
   - （2）　有時候這樣。
   - （3）　只是間中這樣。
   - （4）　沒有這樣。

10. 我想過要傷害自己。
    - （1）　相當多時候這樣
    - （2）　有時候這樣。
    - （3）　很少這樣。
    - （4）　沒有這樣。

© The Royal College of Psychiatrists 1987. Translated from Cox JL, Holden JM, Sagovsky R (1987) Detection of postnatal depression. Development of the 10-item Edinburgh Postnatal Depression Scale. *British Journal of Psychiatry*, **150**, 782–786.

Chinese (Taiwan)

恭喜您，您有了寶寶，我們想瞭解您的感受，請仔細閱讀每一個問題，選出最貼近您最近七天的感受的選項（在選項前的空格打勾）。 **範例：**

> 我覺得快樂
> ☐ **a.** 是，一直都是這樣
> ☑ **b.** 是，大部分時間是這樣
> ☐ **c.** 不，不常這樣
> ☐ **d.** 不，一點也沒有

上例中，選 b 表示 "我在過去七天中，大部分時間覺得快樂"
請照同樣方式完成以下各題。*注意：請回答最近七天的感受，不只是今天一天的感受。*

在最近七天中

1. 我能開懷地笑，並看到事物有趣的一面
☐ a.跟往常一樣
☐ b.似乎沒有往常那麼多
☐ c.肯定比往常少
☐ d.完全不能

2. 我欣然期待未來的一切
☐ a.跟往常一樣
☐ b.似乎沒有往常那麼多
☐ c.肯定比往常少
☐ d.完全不能

3. 當事情出錯時，我會不必要地責備自己
☐ a.是，大部分時候會
☐ b.是，有時候會
☐ c.不常這樣
☐ d.不，從來不會

4. 我無緣無故地覺得緊張或擔憂
☐ a.不，一點也沒有
☐ b.極少有
☐ c.是，有時候這樣
☐ d.是，常常這樣

5. 我無緣無故地覺得害怕或恐慌
☐ a.是，很多時候這樣
☐ b.是，有時候會這樣
☐ c.不，不常這樣
☐ d.不，一點也不會

6. 事情多得幾乎要壓過我
☐ a.是，大部分時候我已經完全無法應付
☐ b.是，有時候我沒辦法應付得像以前那麼好
☐ c.不會，大部分時候我應付得還不錯
☐ d.不會，我一直都能應付得好

7. 我很不快樂，以致於睡不好
☐ a.是，大部分時候都這樣
☐ b.是，有時候這樣
☐ c.不常這樣
☐ d.不，一點也不會

8. 我感到難過或悲哀
☐ a.是，大部分時候這樣
☐ b.是，很常這樣
☐ c.不常這樣
☐ d.不，一點也不會

9. 我覺得很不快樂而哭泣
☐ a.是，大部分時候這樣
☐ b.是，很常這樣
☐ c.只有偶爾這樣
☐ d.不，從來沒有

10. 我想過要傷害自己
☐ a.是，常常
☐ b.有時候
☐ c.幾乎沒有
☐ d.從來沒有

Czech

Jak se cítíte?

Poněvadž se Vám nedávno narodilo dítě, rádi bychom se Vás zeptali, jak se nyní cítíte. Podškrtněte prosím tu odpověď, která nejlépe vyjádřuje Vaše pocity během posledních 7 dnů, ne jenom to jak se cítíte dnes. Zde je již hotový příklad:

Cítila jsem se šťastná:

    Ano, většinu času

    <u>Ano, někdy</u>

    Ne, ne příliš

    Ne, vůbec ne

To by znamenalo: „Během posledního týdne jsem občas byla šťastná."

Stejným způsobem odpovězte prosím i na další otázky.

Během posledních 7 dnů

1. Byla jsem schopna se smát a vidět věci i z jejich veselé stránky:

    Stejně jako dříve

    Ne tak často jako dříve

    Rozhodně ne tak často jako dříve

    Vůbec ne

2. Těšila jsem se na různé věci:

    Stejně jako dříve

    Poněkud méně než dříve

    Rozhodně méně než dříve

    Téměř vůbec ne

3. Zbytečně jsem si vyčítala, když se něco nepovedlo:

    Ano, většinu času

    Ano, někdy

    Ne příliš často

    Ne, nikdy

4. Bezdůvodně jsem byla znepokojená nebo jsem si dělala obavy:

    Ne, vůbec ne

    Téměř nikdy

    Ano, někdy

    Ano, hodně často

5. Bezdůvodně jsem měla strach nebo jsem zpanikařila:

    Ano, často

    Ano, někdy

    Ne, ne příliš

    Ne, vůbec ne

6. Věci mě přerůstaly přes hlavu:

    Ano, většinu času jsem se vůbec nedovedla vypořádat se situací

    Ano, někdy jsem se nedovedla zcela vypořádat se situací

    Ne, většinu času jsem se docela dobře dovedla vypořádat se situací

    Ne, dovedla jsem se vypořádat se situací stejně jako jindy

7. Byla jsem tak nešťastná, že jsem měla potíže se spánkem:
    Ano, většinu času
    Ano, hodně často
    Ne příliš často
    Ne, nikdy

8. Byla jsem smutná nebo sklíčená:
    Ano, většinu času
    Ano, hodně často
    Ne příliš často
    Ne, vůbec ne

9. Byla jsem tak nešťastná, že jsem plakávala:
    Ano, většinu času
    Ano, hodně často
    Pouze zřídka
    Ne, nikdy

10. Napadla mne myšlenka na sebeublížení:
    Ano, hodně často
    Někdy
    Téměř nikdy
    Nikdy

Dari

۱.در هفت روز گذشته، من به توانسته ام خنده کنم و قسمت خنده دار چیز ها را بفهمم:

☐ به همان اندازه که همیشه می توانستم
☐ در حال حاضر نه خیلی زیاد
☐ قطعاً، نه زیاد در حال حاضر
☐ اصلاً

۲. در هفت روز گذشته، من به به آینده خوش بین بوده ام: (امید آینده خوش دارم)

☐ به همان اندازه که تا حالا بوده ام
☐ نسبتاً کمتر از آنچه که قبلاً بوده ام
☐ قطعاً کمتر از آنچه قبلا بوده ام
☐ تقریباً اصلاً

۳. در هفت روز گذشته، وقتی کاری غلط می شد، بدون کدام دلیل خودم را ملامت کرده ام: (گناهکار احساس کرده ام)

☐ بله، زیادتر وقت ها
☐ بله، بعضی وقت ها
☐ نه زیادتر وقت ها
☐ نه، هرگز

۴. در هفت روز گذشته، بدون هیچ کدام دلیل خوبی احساس نگرانی و تشویش کرده ام: (پریشان شده ام)

☐ نه، اصلاً
☐ خیلی کم (یگان وقتی)
☐ بله، بعضی اوقات
☐ بله، زیادتر وقت ها

۵. در هفت روز گذشته، بدون هیچ کدام دلیل خوبی احساس ترس و واهمه داشته ام (دلم می لرزد):

☐ بله، خیلی زیاد
☐ بله، بعضی اوقات
☐ نه، نه زیاد
☐ نه، اصلاً

6. در هفت روز گذشته، همه چیز برام سخت شده است:

بله، زیادتر وقت ها اصلاً نتوانسته ام از عهده کارها بر بیایم ☐
بله، بعضی وقت ها نتوانستم به خوبی همیشه از عهده کارها بر بیایم ☐
نه، زیادتر وقت ها به خوبی از عهده کارها بر آمده ام ☐
نه، به خوبی همیشه از عهده کارها بر آمده ام ☐

7. در هفت روز گذشته، آنقدر ناراحت بوده ام که مشکل خواب می کردم: (خوابم خراب شده)

بله، زیادتر وقت ها ☐
بله، بعضی اوقات ☐
نه زیاد تر وقت ها ☐
نه، اصلاً ☐

8. در هفت روز گذشته، احساس غمگینی و درماندگی کرده ام: (جگر خونی، بی کسی و تنهایی)

بله، زیادتر وقت ها ☐
بله، نسبتاً اغلب وقت ها ☐
نه زیادتر وقت ها ☐
نه، اصلاً ☐

9. در هفت روز گذشته، چنان ناراحت بوده ام که گریه کرده ام:

بله، زیادتر وقت ها ☐
بله، نسبتاً اغلب وقت ها ☐
فقط گاهگاهی (یگان وقتی) ☐
نه، هرگز ☐

10. در هفت روز گذشته، به فکر این بوده ام که بلایی سر خودم بیاورم:

بله، نسبتاً اغلب وقت ها ☐
بعضی وقت ها ☐
کمتر (یگان وقتی) ☐
هرگز ☐

Dutch

Hoe voelt u zich?

Aangezien u onlangs een baby heeft gehad willen wij graag weten hoe u zich nu voelt. <u>Onderstreep</u> aub het antwoord dat het beste beschrijft hoe u zich de laatste 7 dagen heeft gevoeld, niet alleen hoe u zich vandaag voelt. Hieronder volgt een voorbeeld:

> Ik voel me gelukkig:
> Ja, over het algemeen
> <u>Ja, soms</u>
> Nee, niet echt
> Nee, helemaal niet

In dit geval zou uw antwoord betekenen: 'Ik heb me soms gelukkig gevoeld in de afgelopen week'. Beantwoord aub de volgende vragen op dezelfde manier.

In de afgelopen 7 dagen

1. Ik heb kunnen lachen en de zonnige kant van de dingen kunnen inzien:
   Zoveel als ik altijd kon
   Niet zo veel nu als anders
   Zeker niet zo veel nu als anders
   Helemaal niet

2. Ik heb met plezier naar dingen uitgekeken:
   Zoals altijd of meer
   Wat minder dan ik gewend was
   Absoluut minder dan ik gewend was
   Nauwelijks

3. Ik heb mij zelf onnodig verwijten gemaakt als er iets fout ging:
   Ja, heel vaak
   Ja, soms
   Niet erg vaak
   Nee, nooit

4. Ik ben bang of bezorgd geweest zonder dat er een aanleiding was:
   Nee, helemaal niet
   Nauwelijks
   Ja, soms
   Ja, zeer vaak

5. Ik reageerde schrikachtig of paniekerig zonder echt goede reden:
   Ja, tamelijk vaak
   Ja, soms
   Nee, niet vaak
   Nooit

6. De dingen groeiden me boven het hoofd:
   Ja, meestal was ik er niet tegen opgewassen
   Ja, soms was ik minder goed tegen dingen opgewassen dan anders
   Nee, meestal kon ik de dingen erg goed aan
   Nee, ik kon alles even goed aan als anders

7. Ik voelde me zo ongelukkig dat ik er bijna niet van kon slapen:
   Ja, meestal
   Ja, soms
   Niet vaak
   Helemaal niet

8. Ik voelde me somber en beroerd:
   Ja, bijna steeds
   Ja, tamelijk vaak
   Niet erg vaak
   Nee, helemaal niet

9. Ik was zo ongelukkig dat ik heb zitten huilen:
   Ja, heel vaak
   Ja, tamelijk vaak
   Alleen af en toe
   Nee, nooit

10. Ik heb era aan gedacht om mezelf iets aan te doen:
    Ja, tamelijk vaak
    Soms
    Nauwelijks
    Nooit

Estonian

Kuna te ootate last või olete hiljuti sünnitanud, soovime teada, kuidas te end tunnete. Palun märkige ära vastus, mis on lähim sellele, kuidas te end **viimase 7 päeva jooksul**, mitte ainult täna, tundsite.

Siin on üks vastatud näide

Olen tundnud end õnnelikuna:
Jah, kogu aeg
Jah, enamus ajast (See võiks tähendada 'Ma olen olnud õnnelik enamus ajast' viimase nädala jooksul)
Ei, mitte väga tihti
Ei, üldse mitte   Palun täitke teised küsimused samal moel.

Viimase 7 päeva jooksul

1. Olen olnud võimeline naerma ja nägema asjade toredat külge:
   Sama palju kui alati
   Praegu veidi vähem
   Praegu tunduvalt vähem
   Üldse mitte

2. Olen oodanud asju rõõmuga:
   Sama palju kui varem
   Pigem vähem kui tavaliselt
   Kindlasti vähem kui tavaliselt
   Üldse mitte

3. Olen end asjatult süüdistanud, kui asjad on läinud valesti:
   Jah, enamus ajast
   Jah, mõnikord
   Mitte eriti sageli
   Ei, mitte kunagi

4. Olen olnud ärev või muretsenud ilma erilise põhjuseta:
   Ei, üldse mitte
   Harva
   Jah, mõnikord
   Jah, väga sageli

5. Olen tundnud hirmu või paanikat ilma erilise põhjuseta:
   Jah, üsna palju
   Jah, mõnikord
   Ei, mitte kuigi palju
   Ei, üldse mitte

6. Asjad on mul üle pea kasvanud:
   Jah, enamus ajast ma ei tule üldse toime
   Jah, mõnikord ma ei tule nii hästi toime kui tavaliselt
   Ei, enamus ajast tulen toime küllalt hästi
   Ei, tulen toime sama hästi kui alati

7. Olen olnud nii õnnetu, et mul on olnud raskusi magamisega:
   Jah, enamus ajast
   Jah, küllalt sageli
   Mitte eriti sageli
   Ei, üldse mitte

8. Olen tundnud kurbust ja masendust:
   Jah, enamus ajast
   Jah, küllalt sageli
   Mitte eriti sageli
   Ei, üldse mitte

9. Olen olnud nii õnnetu, et olen nutnud:
   Jah, enamus ajast
   Jah, küllalt sageli
   Ainult vahetevahel
   Ei, mitte kunagi

10. Mul on esinenud mõtteid enese vigastamisest:
    Jah, küllalt sageli
    Mõnikord
    Peaaegu mitte kunagi
    Mitte kordagi

Farsi/Persian

چه احساسی دارید؟

باین دلیل که شما به تازگی زایمان نموده اید، ما علاقمندیم بدانیم در حال حاضر چه احساسی دارید. لطفا زیر جوابی را که نمایش خط بکشید.

دهنده احساس شما، نه فقط در حال حاضر بلکه در هفت روز گذشته می باشد، _____ این یك نمونه از سئوالها است که جواب داده شده است:

من احساس شادی کرده ام:
بله، اکثر اوقات
بله، گاهی اوقات
خیر، نه زیاد
خیر، ابدا

که بدین معنی است : " من در طول هفته گذشته گاهی اوقات احساس خوشحالی کرده ام"

لطفا باقی سئوالات را به همین طریق کامل نمائید.

در هفت روز گذشته:

1 - توانستم بخندم و طنز را در مسائل به بینم:
بهمان اندازه که همیشه می توانستم
در حال حاضر نه چندان
بطور قطع در حال حاضر نمی توانم
ابدا

2 - با لذت در انتظار اتفاقات روزمره بوده ام :
بهمان اندازه که همیشه لذت می بردم
تقریبا کمتر از آنچه عادت داشتم
مطمئنا کمتر از گذشته
ابدا

3 - وقتی که مسائل بدرستی پیش نمیروند خودم را سرزنش کرده ام:
بله، اکثر اوقات
بله، گاهی اوقات
در اکثر اوقات، خیر
خیر، هرگز

(لطفا به سئوالات 4 - 10 در پشت این صفحه پاسخ دهید)

4 - بدون دلیل نگران و مضطرب بوده ام:
خیر، ابدا
خیلی بندرت
بله، گاهی اوقات
بله، اغلب اوقات

5 - بدون دلیل خاص احساس ترس و وحشت کرده ام:
بله، خیلی زیاد
بله، گاهی اوقات
خیر، نه زیاد
خیر، ابدا

6 - مسائل بر من غلبه میکنند:
بله، اکثر اوقات نتوانسته ام با مسائل بخوبی مواجه شوم
بله، گاهی اوقات نتوانسته ام مانند سابق با مسائل برخورد نمایم
خیر، اغلب اوقات بخوبی توانسته ام از عهده مسائل بر آیم
خیر، مانند همیشه با مسائل کنار آمده ام

7 - بله، اکثر اوقات افسردگی من بقدری شدید بوده که باعث بیخوابی شده است:
بله، اغلب
خیر، خیلی بندرت
خیر، ابدا

8 - من احساس غم و بیچاره گی کرده ام:
بله، اکثر اوقات
بله، اغلب
اکثرا خیر
خیر، ابدا

9 - میزان غم و اندوه ام آنقدر زیاد بوده که گریه کرده ام:
بله، اکثر اوقات
بله اغلب
فقط گاهی اوقات
خیر، هرگز

10 - فکر صدمه زدن بخودم به مغزم خطور کرده است:
اغلب اوقات
گاهی اوقات
خیلی بندرت
هرگز

Filipino/Tagalog

Kumusta na ang iyong pakiramdam?

Sa dahilang ikaw ay nanganak kamakailan lamang, nais naming malaman kung ano ang iyong pakiramdam sa ngayon. Mangyari lamang na guhitan ang sagot na pinakamalapit sa iyong naramdaman sa nakaraang 7 araw, hindi lamang ang iyong nararamdaman sa ngayon. Narito ang isang halimbawa, na nasagutan na:

> Ako ay nakaramdam ng kaligayahan:
> Oo, kadalasan
> Oo, minsan
> Hindi, hindi gaano
> Hindi, hindi ni minsan

Nangangahulugan ito na: 'Minsan ako ay nakaramdam ng kaligayan sa nakaraang linggo'. Mangyari lamang na kumpletohin ang iba pang mga katanungan sa parehong paraan.

Sa nakaraang 7 araw

1. Nagawa kong tumawa at nakita ko ang nakakatuwang bahagi ng mga bagay:
   Kasing dalas ng palagi kong ginagawa
   Hindi na gaano kadalas sa ngayon
   Talagang hindi na gaano kadalas sa ngayon
   Hindi ni minsan

2. Umaasa ako na masisiyahan sa mga bagay:
   Kasing dalas ng dati kong ginagawa
   Hindi na gaano kadalas katulad ng dati kong ginagawa
   Talagang di na gaano kadalas katulad ng dati kong ginagawa
   Bibihirang mangyari

3. Sinisi ko ang aking sarili kapag may mga maling bagay na nangyari:
   Oo, kadalasan
   Oo, minsan
   Hindi gaanong madalas
   Hindi, hindi kailanman

4. Nag-alala ako o nabalisa nang walang magandang kadahilanan:
   Hindi, hindi ni minsan
   Bibihirang mangyari
   Oo, kung minsan
   Oo, napakadalas

5. Nakaramdam ako ng takot o biglang pagkatakot nang walang magandang dahilan:
   Oo, napakadalas
   Oo, paminsan-minsan
   Hindi, hindi gaanong madalas
   Hindi, hindi ni minsan

6. Nahihirapan akong makayanan ang mga bagay:
   Oo, kadalasan ay hindi ko nakakayanan ang mga bagay
   Oo, paminsan-minsan ay hindi ko nakakayanan ang mga bagay nang kasing husay ng dati
   Hindi, kadalasan ay nakayanan ko nang mahusay ang mga bagay
   Hindi, nakakayanan ko ang mga bagay katulad ng palagian

7. Naging sobrang malungkutin ako kaya nahirapan ako sa pagtulog:
   Oo, kadalasan
   Oo, napakadalas
   Hindi gaanong madalas
   Hindi, hindi kailanman

8. Nakaramdam ako ng lungkot at pagiging kahabag-habag:
   Oo, kadalasan
   Oo, napakadalas
   Hindi gaanong madalas
   Hindi, kailanma'y hindi

9. Naging malungkutin ako na naging dahilan ng aking pag-iyak:
   Oo, kadalasan
   Oo, napakadalas
   Paminsan-minsan lamang
   Hindi, kailanma'y hindi

10. Ang pag-iisip na saktan ang aking sarili ay nangyari sa akin:
    Oo, napakadalas
    Paminsan-minsan
    Bibihirang mangyari
    Hindi kailanman

Finnish

Ole hyvä ja ympyröi vaihtoehto, joka parhaiten vastaa Sinun tuntemuksiasi viimeisen kuluneen viikon aikana, ei vain tämänhetkisiä tuntemuksiasi.

Viimeisten seitsemän päivän aikana

1. olen pystynyt nauramaan ja näkemään asioiden hauskan puolen
   yhtä paljon kuin aina ennenkin
   en aivan yhtä paljon kuin ennen
   selvästi vähemmän kuin ennen
   en ollenkaan

2. olen odotellut mielihyvällä tulevia tapahtumia
   yhtä paljon kuin aina ennenkin
   hiukan vähemmän kuin aikaisemmin
   selvästi vähemmän kuin aikaisemmin
   tuskin lainkaan

3. olen syyttänyt tarpeettomasti itseäni, kun asiat ovat menneet vikaan
   kyllä, useimmiten
   kyllä, joskus
   en kovin usein
   en koskaan

4. olen ollut ahdistunut tai huolestunut ilman selvää syytä
   ei, en ollenkaan
   tuskin koskaan
   kyllä, joskus
   kyllä, hyvin usein

5. olen ollut peloissani tai hädissäni ilman erityistä selvää syytä
   kyllä, aika paljon
   kyllä, joskus
   ei, en paljonkaan
   ei, en ollenkaan

6. asiat kasautuvat päälleni
   kyllä, useimmiten en ole pystynyt selviytymään niistä ollenkaan
   kyllä, toisinaan en ole selviytynyt niistä yhtä hyvin kuin tavallisesti
   ei, useimmiten olen selviytynyt melko hyvin
   ei, olen selviytynyt niistä yhtä hyvin kuin aina ennenkin

7. olen ollut niin onneton, että minulla on ollut univaikeuksia
   kyllä, useimmiten
   kyllä, toisinaan
   ei, en kovin usein
   ei, en ollenkaan

8. olen tuntenut oloni surulliseksi ja kurjaksi
   kyllä, useimmiten
   kyllä, melko usein
   en kovin usein
   ei, en ollenkaan

9. olen ollut niin onneton, että olen itkeskellyt
   kyllä, useimmiten
   kyllä, melko usein
   vain silloin tällöin
   ei, en koskaan

10. ajatus itseni vahingoittamisesta on tullut mieleeni
    kyllä, melko usein
    joskus
    tuskin koskaan
    ei koskaan

Kysymyksissä 1, 2 ja 4 vastausvaihtoehdot pisteytetään järjestyksessä ylimmästä alimpaan asteikolla 0–3. Kysymykset 3 sekä 5–10 ovat käänteisiä ja ne pisteytetään järjestyksessä ylimmästä alimpaan asteikolla 3–0.

EPDS-mittari on validoitu useassa maassa, eikä sitä saa toimipaikkakohtaisesti muuttaa.

French

Vous venez d'avoir un bébé. Nous aimerions savoir comment vous vous sentez. Nous vous demandons de bien vouloir remplir ce questionnaire en soulignant la réponse qui vous semble le mieux décrire comment vous vous êtes sentie durant la semaine (c'est-à-dire sur les 7 jours qui viennent de s'écouler) et pas seulement au jour d'aujourd'hui:

Voici un exemple

> Je me suis sentie heureuse:
> Oui, tout le temps
> <u>Oui, la plupart du temps</u>
> Non, pas très souvent
> Non, pas du tout.

Ceci signifiera 'je me suis sentie heureuse la plupart du temps durant la semaine qui vient de s'écouler'. Merci de bien vouloir répondre aux autres questions.

Pendant la semaine qui vient de s'ecouler

1. J'ai pu rire et prendre les choses du bon côté:
   Aussi souvent que d'habitude
   Pas tout-à-fait autant
   Vraiment beaucoup moins souvent ces jours-ci
   Absolument pas

2. Je me suis sentie confiante et joyeuse, en pensant à l'avenir:
   Autant que d'habitude
   Plutôt moins que d'habitude
   Vraiment moins que d'habitude
   Pratiquement pas

3. Je me suis reprochée, sans raisons, d'être responsable quand les choses allaient mal:
   Oui, la plupart du temps
   Oui, parfois
   Pas très souvent
   Non, jamais

4. Je me suis sentie inquiète ou soucieuse sans motifs:
   Non, pas du tout
   Presque jamais
   Oui, parfois
   Oui, très souvent

5. Je me suis sentie effrayée ou paniquée sans vraiment de raisons:
   Oui, vraiment souvent
   Oui, parfois
   Non, pas très souvent
   Non, pas du tout

6. J'ai eu tendance à me sentir dépassée par les évènements:
   Oui, la plupart du temps, je me suis sentie incapable de faire face aux situations
   Oui, parfois, je ne me suis pas sentie aussi capable de faire face que d'habitude
   Non, j'ai pu faire face à la plupart des situations
   Non, je me suis sentie aussi efficace que d'habitude

7. Je me suis sentie si malheureuse que j'ai eu des problèmes de sommeil:
   Oui, la plupart du temps
   Oui, parfois
   Pas très souvent
   Non, pas du tout

8. Je me suis sentie triste ou peu heureuse:
   Oui, la plupart du temps
   Oui, très souvent
   Pas très souvent
   Non, pas du tout

9. Je me suis sentie si malheureuse que j'en ai pleuré:
   Oui, la plupart du temps
   Oui, très souvent
   Seulement de temps en temps
   Non, jamais

10. Il m'est arrivé de penser à me faire du mal:
    Oui, très souvent
    Parfois
    Presque jamais
    Jamais

German

Wie fühlen Sie sich?

Da Sie kürzlich ein Baby bekommen haben, möchten wir gerne von Ihnen wissen, wie Sie sich jetzt fühlen. Bitte, unterstreichen Sie diejenige Antwort, die am besten beschreibt, wie Sie sich während der letzten sieben Tage, also nicht nur heute, gefühlt haben: Hier ist ein bereits ausgefülltes Beispiel:

> Ich war glücklich:
> Ja, meistens
> Ja, manchmal
> Nein, nicht sehr oft
> Nein, gar nicht

Das würde bedeuten: ‚Während dieser Woche habe ich mich manchmal glücklich gefühlt.' Bitte beantworten Sie in gleicher Weise auch die übrigen Fragen.

Während der letzten 7 Tage

1. Ich konnte lachen und die komische Seite von Dingen sehen:
   So viel wie bisher
   Nicht ganz wie früher
   Bestimmt nicht so sehr wie bisher
   Überhaupt nicht

2. Ich habe mich auf Dinge im voraus gefreut:
   So viel wie bisher
   Wohl weniger als gewöhnlich
   Bestimmt weniger als gewöhnlich
   Fast nie

3. Ich habe mich schuldig gefühlt, wenn etwas schief ging:
   Ja, meistens
   Ja, manchmal
   Nicht sehr oft
   Nein, nie

4. Ich war ängstlich oder besorgt ohne einen guten Grund:
   Nein, gar nicht
   Kaum jemals
   Ja, manchmal
   Ja, sehr oft

5. Ich habe mich gefürchtet oder war von Panik ergriffen ohne einen guten Grund:
    Ja, sehr häufig
    Ja, manchmal
    Nein, nicht besonders
    Nein, gar nicht

6. Dinge wurden mir einfach zuviel:
    Ja, meistens konnte ich die Situation gar nicht meistern
    Ja, manchmal konnte ich die Situation nicht so gut wie sonst meistern
    Nein, meistens konnte ich die Situation ganz gut meistern
    Nein, ich bewältigte Dinge so gut wie immer

7. Ich war so unglücklich, daß ich nur schlecht schlafen konnte:
    Ja, meistens
    Ja, ziemlich häufig
    Nicht sehr oft
    Nein, nie

8. Ich habe mich traurig oder elend gefühlt:
    Ja, meistens
    Ja, ziemlich häufig
    Nein, nicht sehr häufig
    Nein, gar nicht

9. Ich war so unglücklich, daß ich weinen musste:
    Ja, meistens
    Ja, ziemlich häufig
    Nur gelegentlich
    Nein, nie

10. Der Gedanke, mir etwas anzutun, ist mir eingefallen:
    Ja, ziemlich häufig
    Manchmal
    Kaum jemals
    Niemals

Greek

Πώς αισθάνεστε;
Μετά από την πρόσφατη γέννηση του παιδιού σας, θα θέλαμε να μάθουμε πώς αισθάνεστε τώρα. Παρακαλώ <u>υπογραμμίστε</u> την απάντηση που αντιστοιχεί πλησιέστερα στο πώς αισθανόσαστε τις περασμένες 7 ημέρες, όχι μόνο στο πώς αισθάνεστε σήμερα. Να ένα παράδειγμα, που είναι ήδη συμπληρωμένο:

Αισθανόμουν χαρούμενη:
Ναι, το περισσότερο χρονικό διάστημα
<u>Ναι, μερικό χρονικό διάστημα</u>
Όχι, όχι τόσο πολύ
Όχι, καθόλου

Αυτό θα εννοούσε: «Αισθάνθηκα χαρούμενη για μερικό χρονικό διάστημα κατά την περασμένη εβδομάδα».
Σας παρακαλούμε να συμπληρώσετε τις υπόλοιπες ερωτήσεις κατά τον ίδιο τρόπο.

Τις τελευταίες 7 ημέρες

1. Μπορούσα να γελώ και να βλέπω την αστεία πλευρά της ζωής:
   Όπως πριν
   Λιγότερο από πριν
   Πολύ λιγότερο από πριν
   Καθόλου

2. Έβλεπα το αύριο με ενθουσιασμό:
   Όπως και πριν
   Μάλλον λιγότερο από πριν
   Πολύ λιγότερο από πριν
   Σχεδόν καθόλου

3. Κατηγορούσα άδικα τον εαυτό μου για πράγματα που πήγαν στραβά:
   Ναι, όλη την ώρα
   Ναι, αρκετά συχνά
   Όχι πολύ συχνά
   Όχι, ποτέ

4. Ένιωθα άγχος ή ανησυχία χωρίς σοβαρό λόγο:
   Όχι, καθόλου
   Σχεδόν ποτέ
   Ναι, μερικές φορές
   Ναι, πολύ συχνά

5. Ένιωθα φόβο ή πανικό, χωρίς σοβαρό λόγο:
   Ναι, πολύ συχνά
   Ναι, μερικές φορές
   Όχι, όχι συχνά
   Όχι, καθόλου

6. Με πήρε η κάτω βόλτα (ένιωθα πολύ πεσμένη):
   Ναι, τις περισσότερες φορές δεν ήμουν σε θέση να τα βγάλω πέρα καθόλου
   Ναι, μερικές φορές δεν τα βγάζω πέρα τόσο καλά όσο συνήθως
   Όχι, τις περισσότερες φορές τα έβγαλα πέρα αρκετά καλά
   Όχι, τα βγάζω πέρα καλά, όπως πάντα

7. Ήμουν τόσο στενοχωρημένη που δεν μπορούσα να κοιμηθώ:
   Ναι, σχεδόν συνέχεια
   Ναι, αρκετά συχνά
   Σπάνια
   Όχι, καθόλου

8. Ένιωθα θλιμμένη ή λυπημένη:
   Ναι, σχεδόν συνέχεια
   Ναι, αρκετά συχνά
   Σπάνια
   Όχι, καθόλου

9. Ένιωθα τόσο στενοχωρημένη που έκλαιγα:
   Ναι, όλη την ώρα
   Ναι, αρκετά συχνά
   Κάπου-κάπου
   Όχι, ποτέ

10. Μου ήρθε να βλάψω τον εαυτό μου:
    Ναι, αρκετά συχνά
    Μερικές φορές
    Σχεδόν ποτέ
    Ποτέ

Hebrew

איך את מרגישה?

לא מזמן ילדת את תינוקך, ברצוננו לדעת כיצד את מרגישה כרגע. בבקשה מתחי קו מתחת לתשובה הכי מתאימה המביעה את הרגשתך בשבעה ימים האחרונים, לא רק מה שאת מרגישה היום.

להלן תמצאי דוגמא שהכנו עבורך:

הרגשתי שמחה:

כן, רב הזמן
<u>כן, חלק מהזמן</u>
לא, לא כל כך
לא, בכלל לא

זה אומר: 'הרגשתי שמחה בחלק מהזמן במשך השבוע האחרון'

בבקשה השלימי את שאר השאלות באותה צורה.

בשבעה ימים האחרונים

1. הייתי מסוגלת לצחוק ולראות את הצד המצחיק של דברים.
   כפי שיכולתי תמיד
   פחות מתמיד
   הרבה פחות מתמיד
   בכלל לא

2. ציפיתי בהנאה לדברים שיקרו.
   כפי שיכולתי תמיד
   פחות משהייתי רגילה
   הרבה פחות משהייתי רגילה
   כמעט בכלל לא

3. האשמתי את עצמי שלא לצורך כאשר דברים לא הסתדרו.
   כן, רוב הזמן
   כן, חלק מהזמן
   לעיתים רחוקות
   אף פעם

4. הרגשתי חרדה או דאגה ללא כל סיבה.
   בכלל לא
   לעיתים רחוקות
   כן, לפעמים
   כן, לעיתים קרובות מאוד

5. הרגשתי מפוחדת או מבוהלת ללא כל סיבה מוצדקת.
   כן, לעיתים קרובות
   כן, לפעמים
   לעיתים רחוקות
   בכלל לא

6. הרגשתי שדברים קשים לי מדי.
   כן, לרוב לא יכולתי להתמודד בכלל
   כן, לפעמים לא יכולתי להתמודד כפי שאני רגילה
   לא, בדרך כלל התמודדתי (הסתדרתי) די טוב
   לא, אני מתמודדת כמו תמיד

7. הרגשתי כה אומללה שהיה לי קשה לישון.
   כן, בדרך כלל
   כן, לפעמים
   לעיתים רחוקות
   בכלל לא

8. הרגשתי עצובה או אומללה (מצוברחת).
   כן רוב הזמן
   כן, לעיתים קרובות
   לעיתים רחוקות
   בכלל לא

9. הרגשתי כה אומללה שבכיתי.
   רוב הזמן
   לעיתים קרובות
   מדי פעם
   בכלל לא

10. המחשבה לפגוע בעצמי עלתה בראשי.
    כן, לעיתים קרובות
    לפעמים
    כמעט לא
    בכלל לא

Hindi

Kumusta na ang iyong pakiramdam?

Sa dahilang ikaw ay nanganak kamakailan lamang, nais naming malaman kung ano ang iyong pakiramdam sa ngayon. Mangyari lamang na guhitan ang sagot na pinakamalapit sa iyong naramdaman sa nakaraang 7 araw, hindi lamang ang iyong nararamdaman sa ngayon. Narito ang isang halimbawa, na nasagutan na:

> Ako ay nakaramdam ng kaligayahan:
> Oo, kadalasan
> Oo, minsan
> Hindi, hindi gaano
> Hindi, hindi ni minsan

Nangangahulugan ito na: 'Minsan ako ay nakaramdam ng kaligayan sa nakaraang linggo'. Mangyari lamang na kumpletohin ang iba pang mga katanungan sa parehong paraan.

Sa nakaraang 7 araw

1. Nagawa kong tumawa at nakita ko ang nakakatuwang bahagi ng mga bagay:
   Kasing dalas ng palagi kong ginagawa
   Hindi na gaano kadalas sa ngayon
   Talagang hindi na gaano kadalas sa ngayon
   Hindi ni minsan

2. Umaasa ako na masisiyahan sa mga bagay:
   Kasing dalas ng dati kong ginagawa
   Hindi na gaano kadalas katulad ng dati kong ginagawa
   Talagang di na gaano kadalas katulad ng dati kong ginagawa
   Bibihirang mangyari

3. Sinisi ko ang aking sarili kapag may mga maling bagay na nangyari:
   Oo, kadalasan
   Oo, minsan
   Hindi gaanong madalas
   Hindi, hindi kailanman

4. Nag-alala ako o nabalisa nang walang magandang kadahilanan:
   Hindi, hindi ni minsan
   Bibihirang mangyari
   Oo, kung minsan
   Oo, napakadalas

5. Nakaramdam ako ng takot o biglang pagkatakot nang walang magandang dahilan:
   Oo, napakadalas
   Oo, paminsan-minsan
   Hindi, hindi gaanong madalas
   Hindi, hindi ni minsan

6. Nahihirapan akong makayanan ang mga bagay:
   Oo, kadalasan ay hindi ko nakakayanan ang mga bagay
   Oo, paminsan-minsan ay hindi ko nakakayanan ang mga bagay nang kasing husay ng dati
   Hindi, kadalasan ay nakayanan ko nang mahusay ang mga bagay
   Hindi, nakakayanan ko ang mga bagay katulad ng palagian

7. Naging sobrang malungkutin ako kaya nahirapan ako sa pagtulog:
   Oo, kadalasan
   Oo, napakadalas
   Hindi gaanong madalas
   Hindi, hindi kailanman

8. Nakaramdam ako ng lungkot at pagiging kahabag-habag:
   Oo, kadalasan
   Oo, napakadalas
   Hindi gaanong madalas
   Hindi, kailanma'y hindi

9. Naging malungkutin ako na naging dahilan ng aking pag-iyak:
   Oo, kadalasan
   Oo, napakadalas
   Paminsan-minsan lamang
   Hindi, kailanma'y hindi

10. Ang pag-iisip na saktan ang aking sarili ay nangyari sa akin:
    Oo, napakadalas
    Paminsan-minsan
    Bibihirang mangyari
    Hindi kailanman

Hungarian

Mivel Ön terhes, vagy mostanában szu¨ letett gyermeke, azt szeretnénk megtudni, hogyan érzi magát. Kérem, jelölje be azokat a válaszokat, amelyek a legközelebb álltak ahhoz, ahogy Ön érezte magát **az elmúlt 7 napban** (és nem csak jelenleg).

Az elmu'lt 7 napban

1. Képes voltam nevetni és a dolgok mulatságos oldalát nézni.
   Ugyanolyan gyakran, mint korábban
   Talán kicsit ritkábban
   Egyértelműen ritkábban
   Egyáltalán nem

2. Örömmel vártam bizonyos dolgokat.
   Ugyanúgy, mint régen
   Talán kicsit ritkábban
   Egyértelműen ritkábban
   Egyáltalán nem

3. Feleslegesen hibáztattam magam, amikor a dolgok rosszul mentek.
   Többnyire igen
   Elég gyakran
   Nem túl gyakran
   Soha

4. Minden különösebb ok nélkül szorongóvá, aggodalmassá váltam.
   Soha
   Kivételes esetekben
   Több alkalommal
   Nagyon gyakran

5. Minden különösebb ok nélkül félelem vagy pánik tört rám.
   Nagyon gyakran
   Több alkalommal
   Kivételes esetekben
   Soha

6. Összecsaptak fejem fölött a hullámok.
   Igen, többnyire nem tudtam megbirkózni a dolgokkal.
   Igen, néha nem tudok oly mértékben megbirkózni azokkal, mint korábban.
   Nem, többnyire jól elboldogulok azokkal.
   Nem, ugyanolyan jól megbirkózom azokkal, mint korábban.

7. Olyan boldogtalan voltam, hogy problémám volt az alvással.
    Többnyire igen
    Több alkalommal
    Csak ritkán
    Soha nem fordult elő

8. Szomorúnak vagy szerencsétlennek éreztem magam.
    Többnyire igen
    Elég gyakran
    Csak ritkán
    Soha nem fordult elő

9. Annyira boldogtalannak éreztem magam, hogy sírva fakadtam.
    Igen, legtöbbször
    Igen, elég gyakran
    Csak ritkán
    Soha nem fordult elő

10. Eszembe jutott már, hogy kárt teszek magamban.
    Elég gyakran
    Néha
    Szinte soha
    Soha

Icelandic

Með eftirfarandi spurningalista er verið að kanna líðan kvenna eftir barnsborð. Vinsamlegast krossaðu framan við það svar sem kemst naest því að lýsa hvernig pér hefur liðið síðastliðna viku.

Mér hefur liðið þnnig síðastliðna viku

1. Ég hef getað hlegið og séð broslegu hliðarnar à lífinu
    Eins mikið og àður
    Ekki alveg eins mikið og àður
    Alls ekki eins mikið og àður
    Alls ekki

2. Ég hlakkaði til ýmissa atburða
    Alveg eins mikið og àður
    Aðeins minna en àður
    Mun minna en àður
    Varla nokkurn tímann

3. Ég hef àsakað sjàlfa mig að ósekju þegar eitthvað fór úrskeiðis
    Jà, jfirleitt
    Jà, stundum
    Sjaldan
    Nei, aldrei

4. Ég hef verið kvíðin og àhyggjufull þó ég hafi ekki haft àstaeðu til
    Nei, alls ekki
    Naestum aldrei
    Jà, stundum
    Jà, mjög oft

5. Ég hef verið hraedd eða strekkt à taugum þó ég hafi ekki haft àstaeðu til
    Jà, nokkuð oft
    Jà, stundum
    Nei, sjaldan
    Nei, aldrei

6. Allt hefur vaxið mér yfir höfuð
    Jà, oftast hef ég ekki getað ràðið við neitt
    Jà, stundum hefur mér gengið verr en vanalega
    Nei, yfirleitt hefur allt gengið vel
    Nei, ég hef ràðið við hlutina eins og venjulega

7. Ég hef verið svo vansael að ég hef átt erfitt með svefn
   Já, yfirleitt
   Já, stundum
   Sjaldan
   Nei, alls ekki

8. Ég hef verið döpur og aum
   Já, naer alltaf
   Já, frekar oft
   Sjaldan
   Nei, alls ekki

9. Ég hef verið svo vansael að ég hef grátið
   Já, mjög oft
   Já, stundum
   Einstaka sinnum
   Nei, aldrei

10. Mér hefur dottið í hug að gera sjàlfri mér mein
    Já, nokkuð oft
    Stundum
    Naer aldrei
    Aldrei

Igbo

Anyi mara na imuru nwa n'isi nso a, o ga – amasi anyi imara otu onodu gi si di. Aziza gig a egosi, obughi nani otu I di taa, ka ma otu onodu si wee diri gi ka mgbe abali asaa gara aga.

> Dika ihe atu: Enwere m obi anuri:
> (a) Oge nile.
> (b) <u>Ee, ihe di ka otutu oge</u>
> (c) Ee e obughi oge nile
> (d) Ee e enweghi m ma - oli

Nke a putara: N'ime abali asaa gara aga, enwere m obi anuri ihe dika otutu oge.

Ugbua, zaa ajuju ndia

1. Enwere m ike ichi ochi, na kwa ihu ihe uto nke ihe:
   (a) Dika m n'emeburi
   (b) Obughi n'uzo di ukuu ugbua
   (c) Odoro anya n'odighi ukuu ugbua
   (d) Odighi ma - oli

2. Ana m ene anya n'ihu inweta ihe uto na - ndu:
   (a) Dika m si enwebu ri
   (b) Opekariri out m si enwebu
   (c) Odoro anya na opekariri nnoo out o na - adiburi
   (d) O n'esi nnoo ike inwe

3. Ana m ata onwe m uta n'uzo n'enweghi isi mgbe ihe anaghi agazi ofuma:
   (a) Ee ihe dika oge nile
   (b) Ee, mgbe ufodu
   (c) Obughi oge nile
   (d) Ee e, odighi mgbe obula nke a n'eme

4. Ana m enwe mgbakasi ah una nchekasi n'uzo n'enweghi isi; (n'enweghi ezi ihe mere ka o di out ahu):
   (a) E e odighi ma - oli
   (b) Nke a n'esi ike ime
   (c) Ee, mgbe ufodu
   (d) Ee, ihe dika oge nile

5. Ujo na mmawapu obi n'enweghi isi turu m mgbe o n'enweghi ezi ihe kpatara ya:
    (a) Ee, o n'eme otutu
    (b) Ee, mgbe ufodu
    (c) Ee e onaghi emesi ike otu ahu
    (d) Ee e onaghi eme ma - oli

6. O di ka-agasi n'ihe nile na-adakwasi m nnoo:
    (a) Ee, ihe kariri otutu ugbo anaghi m enwe ike ma oli inagide ihe omume
    (b) Ee, mgbe ufodu enweghi m ike inagide ihe omume otu m si emebu
    (c) Ee e, otutu mgbe ana m enwe ike inagide ihe omume nke - oma
    (d) Ee e, ana m anagide nnoo ihe omume dika m si eme buri

7. Obi adighi m uto, nke mere n'irahu ura n'esiri m ike:
    (a) Ee ihe dika oge nile
    (b) Ee, mgbe ufodu
    (c) Obughi oge nile
    (d) Ee, e odighi ma - oli

8. Enwere m iwe, obi adighikwa, m uto:
    (a) Ee ihe dika oge nile
    (b) Ee, otutu oge
    (c) Obughi oge nile
    (d) Ee e, odighi ma - oli

9. Ana m ebe nnoo akwa n'ihi na obi adighi m mma:
    (a) Ee ihe dika oge nile
    (b) Ee, otutu oge
    (c) O bun ani odikata
    (d) Ee e, odighi ma - oli

10. O n'abia m n'obi ka mmeru o onwe m ahu:
    (a) Ee, ihe dika oge nile
    (b) Mgbe ufodu
    (c) O n'esi ike
    (d) O dighi ma - oli

Indonesian

Bagaimana perasaan Anda?

Karena Anda baru melahirkan, kami ingin mengetahui bagaimana perasaan Anda sekarang. Silakan menggaris-bawahi jawaban yang paling mirip dengan perasaan Anda selama 7 hari terakhir, tidak hanya perasaan Anda hari ini. Berikut adalah satu contoh yang sudah dijawab:

> Saya merasa senang:
> Ya, hampir terus-menerus
> Ya, kadang-kadang
> Tidak, tidak terlalu
> Tidak sama sekali

Hal ini dapat berarti: 'Sepanjang minggu lalu, saya sering merasa senang'. Silakan menjawab pertanyaan-pertanyaan berikut sebagaimana di atas.

Selama 7 hari terakhir

1. Saya dapat tertawa dan melihat segi kelucuan hal-hal tertentu:
   Seperti biasanya
   Sekarang tidak terlalu sering
   Sekarang agak jarang
   Tidak sama sekali

2. Saya menanti-nanti untuk melakukan sesuatu dengan penuh harapan:
   Hampir seperti biasanya
   Agak berkurang dari biasanya
   Jelas kurang dari biasanya
   Hampir tidak sama sekali

3. Saya menyalahkan diri sendiri jika ada sesuatu yang tidak berjalan dengan baik:
   Ya, hampir selalu
   Ya, kadang-kadang
   Tidak terlalu sering
   Tidak pernah

4. Saya merasa kuatir atau berdebar-debar tanpa alasan:
   Tidak, tidak sama sekali
   Hampir tidak pernah
   Ya, kadang-kadang
   Ya, amat sering

5. Saya merasa takut atau panik tanpa alasan:
   Ya, sering sekali
   Ya, kadang-kadang
   Tidak, tidak terlalu
   Tidak, tidak pernah sama sekali

6. Banyak hal menjadi beban untuk saya:
   Ya, sering kali saya sama sekali tidak dapat mengatasinya
   Ya, kadang saya tidak dapat mengatasi seperti biasanya
   Tidak, biasanya saya dapat mengatasinya dengan baik
   Tidak, saya dapat mengatasinya dengan baik seperti biasanya

7. Saya merasa tidak senang sehingga sukar tidur:
   Ya, hampir selalu
   Ya, sering
   Tidak, tidak sering
   Tidak, tidak pernah

8. Saya merasa sedih atau susah:
   Ya, hampir selalu
   Ya, sering
   Jarang
   Tidak pernah

9. Saya merasa sangat tidak senang menjadikan saya sering menangis:
   Ya, hampir selalu
   Ya, sering
   Hanya sekali-kali
   Tidak pernah

10. Pikiran untuk mencelakai diri sendiri sering muncul:
    Ya, agar sering
    Kadang-kadang
    Hampir tidak pernah
    Tidak pernah

Italian

Lei di recente ha avuto un bambino. Ci piacerebbe sapere come si è sentita nell'ultima settimana. La preghiamo di sottolineare la risposta che meglio descrive come si è sentita nei <u>sette giorni appena trascorsi</u> e non soltanto come si sente oggi. Per aiutarla, ecco un esempio già completato:

> Sono stata felice:
> Sì, sempre
> <u>Sì, per la maggior parte del tempo</u>
> No, non molto spesso
> No, per niente

Il che in pratica significa 'Sono stata per lo più felice durante la scorsa settimana'. Per favor completi le altre domande nello stesso modo.

Nei sette giorni appena trascorsi

1. Sono stata capace di ridere e di vedere il lato comico delle cose:
   Come al solito
   Un po' meno del solito
   Decisamente meno del solito
   Per niente

2. Ho pregustato con piacere le cose:
   Come al solito
   Un po' meno del solito
   Decisamente meno del solito
   A mala pena

3. Ho dato inutilmente la colpa a me stessa quando le cose sono andate male:
   Sì, il più delle volte
   Sì, qualche volta
   Non molto spesso
   No, mai

4. Sono stata ansiosa o preoccupata senza una valida ragione:
   No, per niente
   Quasi mai
   Sì, talvolta
   Sì, spesso

5. Ho provato paura o sono stata in preda al panico senza una valida regione:
   Sì, quasi sempre
   Sì, talvolta
   No, non molto spesso
   Mai

6. Le cose mi hanno causato eccessiva preoccupazione:
   Sì, il più delle volte non sono stata capace di affrontarle
   Sì, qualche volta non sono stata capace di affrontarle come sempre
   No, il più delle volte le ho affrontate abbastanza bene
   No, le ho affrontate bene come sempre

7. Sono stata così infelice che ho avuto difficoltà a dormire:
   Sì, il più delle volte
   Sì, qualche volta
   Non molto spesso
   No, per nulla

8. Mi sono sentita triste o avvilita:
   Sì, per la maggior parte del tempo
   Sì, abbastanza spesso
   Solo occasionalmente
   No, mai

9. Sono stata così infelice che ho pianto:
   Sì, per la maggior parte del tempo
   Sì, abbastanza spesso
   Solo occasionalmente
   No, mai

10. Mi è venuta in mente l'idea di farmi del male:
    Sì, abbastanza spesso
    Qualche volta
    Quasi mai
    Mai

Japanese

エジンバラ産後うつ病調査　　票

ご出産おめでとうございます。ご出産から今までの間にどのようにお感じになったかをお知らせください。今日だけでなく、過去7日間にあなたが感じられたことに最も近い答えにアンダーラインを引いて下さい。必ず10項目に答えてください。

例）　幸せだと感じた。　　　はい、常にそうだった
　　　　　　　　　　　　　はい、たいていそうだった
　　　　　　　　　　　　　いいえ、あまり度々ではなかった
　　　　　　　　　　　　　いいえ、全くそうではなかった

"はい、たいていそうだった"と答えた場合は、過去7日間のことをいいます。この様な方法で質問にお答えください。

【質問】

1. 笑うことができたし、物事のおかしい面もわかった。

　　　　　　　　　　　いつもと同様にできた
　　　　　　　　　　　あまりできなかった
　　　　　　　　　　　明らかにできなかった
　　　　　　　　　　　全くできなかった

2. 物事を楽しみにして待った。

　　　　　　　　　　　いつもと同様にできた
　　　　　　　　　　　あまりできなかった
　　　　　　　　　　　明らかにできなかった
　　　　　　　　　　　ほとんどできなかった

3. 物事が悪くいった時、自分を不必要に責めた

　　　　　　　　　　　はい、たいていそうだった
　　　　　　　　　　　はい、時々そうだった
　　　　　　　　　　　いいえ、あまり度々ではなかった
　　　　　　　　　　　いいえ、そうではなかった

4. はっきりした理由もないのに不安になったり、心配した。

　　　　　　　　　　　いいえ、そうではなかた
　　　　　　　　　　　ほとんどそうではなかた
　　　　　　　　　　　はい、時々あった
　　　　　　　　　　　はい、しょっちゅうあた

5. はっきりした理由もないのに恐怖に襲われた。

　　　　　　　　　　　はい、しょっちゅうあた
　　　　　　　　　　　はい、時々あった
　　　　　　　　　　　いいえ、めったになかた
　　　　　　　　　　　いいえ、全くなかった

6. することがたくさんあって大変だった。

> はい、たいてい対処できなかた
> はい、いつものようにはうまく対処しなかた
> いいえ、たいていうまく対処した
> いいえ、普段通りに対処した

7. 不幸せなので、眠りにくかった。

> はい、ほとんどいつもそうだた
> はい、ときどきそうだった
> いいえ、あまり度々ではなかた
> いいえ、全くなかった

8. 悲しくなったり、惨めになった。

> はい、たいていそうだっ
> はい、かなりしばしばそうだた
> いいえ、あまり度々ではなかた
> いいえ、全くそうではなかった

9. 不幸せなので、泣けてきた。

> はい、たいていそうだった
> はい、かなりしばしばそうだた
> ほんの時々あった
> いいえ、全くそうではなかった

10. 自分自身を傷つけるという考えが浮かんできた。

> はい、かなりしばしばそうだた
> 時々そうだった
> めったになかた
> 全くなかった

Kannada

ಪ್ರಶ್ನೆ 1.

ಮುಂಚೆ ಒಂದು ವಾರದ ದಿನಗಳು:

1. ನೀವು ಏನಾದರು ತಮಾಷೆ ವಸ್ತು ನೋಡುವಾಗ ಮುಂಚೆತರ ನಗುತ್ತೀರಾ.
   - ಮುಂಚೆತರಾ
   - ಸ್ವಲ್ಪ ಕಡಿಮೆ
   - ಜಾಸ್ತಿ ಕಡಿಮೆ
   - ಇಲ್ಲವೆ ಇಲ್ಲ

2. ಮುಂದೆ ಬರುವ ವಸ್ತುವನ್ನು ನೋಡಿ ಸಂತೋಷ ಪಡುವುದು.
   - ನಾನು ಯಾವಾಗಲು ಮಾಡದೇ ಇರುವುದು
   - ಆದಕ್ಕಿಂತ ಕಡಿಮೆ ಉಪಯೋಗಿಸುವುದು.
   - ಕಡಿಂತವಾಗ ಕಡಿಮೆಗಿಂತ ಉಪಯೋಗಿಸುವುದು.
   - ಇಲ್ಲವೇ ಇಲ್ಲ.

3. ಕಾರಣವಿಲ್ಲದೆ ತಮ್ಮ ನಡೆದಾಗ ನನ್ನ ತಪ್ಪನು ನಾಸೆ 3ಲಮಕೂಳ್ಳತ್ತವೆ.
   - ಹೌದು, ಬಹಳ ನೆಮಯು
   - ಹೌದು, ಕೆಲವು ಸಮಯ.
   - ಇಲ್ಲ, ಕಲವೊಮ್ಮೆ
   - ಇಲ್ಲ, ಇಲ್ಲವೆ ಇಲ್ಲ

4. ಕಾರಣವಿಲ್ಲದೆ ನಾನು ಕಾತರಗೊಳ್ಳುವುದು ಅಥವಾ ಚಿಂತೆ ಪಡುವುದು
   - ಇಲ್ಲ, ಇಲ್ಲವೆ ಇಲ್ಲ,
   - ಅಪರೂಪ
   - ಹೌದು, ಕಲವೊಮ್ಮೆ
   - ಹೌದು, ಯಾವಾಗಲು

5. ಕಾರಣವಿಲ್ಲದೆ ಕಾತರಗೊಳ್ಳುವುದು ಅಥವಾ ಭಯಪಡುವುದು
   - ಹೌದು, ಸ್ವಲ್ಪ ಜಾಸ್ತಿ
   - ಹೌದು, ಕಲವೊಮ್ಮೆ
   - ಇಲ್ಲ, ತುಂಬ ಇಲ್ಲ
   - ಇಲ್ಲ, ಇಲ್ಲವೇ ಇಲ್ಲ.

6. ಕಷ್ಟಗಳು ನನ್ನ ಕೈ ಮೀರಿ ಬಂದಾಗ
    . ಹೌದು, ಬಹಳ ಸಮಯ ನನ್ನ ಕಷ್ಟವನ್ನು ನಾನೇ ಬಗೆಹರಿಸಲು ಆಗುವುದಿಲ್ಲ
    . ಹೌದು ಕಲವ್ಪೊಮ್ಮೆ ಆವರ ಜೊತೆ ವಿಗುವುದಕ್ಕೆ ಆಗುವುದಿಲ್ಲ.
    . ಇಲ್ಲ, ಬಹಳ ಸಮಯ ಆವರ ಜೊತೆ ಸಹಕರಿಸಿದ್ದೇನೆ
    . ಇಲ್ಲ, ನಾನು ಯಾವಾಗಲು ಸಹಕರಿಸುತ್ತೇನೆ.

7. ನಾನು ನಿದ್ದೆ ಮಾಡಲು ಕಷಪಡುತ್ತಿದೆ. ಆದ್ದರಿಂದ ನಾನು ಬಹಳ ಉದ್ವಿಗ್ನಗೊಂಡೆ
    . ಹೌದು, ಬಹಳ ಸಮಯ
    . ಹೌದು, ಕೆಲವು ಸಮಯ
    . ಇಲ್ಲ, ಕಲವ್ಪೊಮ್ಮೆ
    . ಇಲ್ಲ, ಇಲ್ಲವೆ ಇಲ್ಲ

8. ನನ್ನಗೆ ಬಹಳ ಬೇಸರಗೊಂಡಾಗ
    . ಹೌದು, ಬಹಳ ಸಮಯ
    . ಹೌದು, ಸ್ವಲ್ಪ ಸಮಯ
    . ಬಿಟ್ಟು,, ಬಿಟ್ಟು,
    . ಇಲ್ಲವೇ ಇಲ್ಲ

9. ನಾನು ಬಹಳ ಅಳುತ್ತಿದ್ದೆ. ಆದ್ದರಿಂದ ನಾನು ಬಹಳ ಉದ್ವಿಗ್ನಗೊಂಡೆ
    . ಹೌದು, ಬಹಳ ಸಮಯ
    . ಹೌದು, ಸ್ವಲ್ಪ ಸಮಯ
    . ಬಿಟ್ಟು ಬಿಟ್ಟು,
    . ಇಲ್ಲವೇ ಇಲ್ಲ.

10. ನನಗೆ ನಾನೇ ನೋವು ಉಂಟುಮಾಡಿಕೊಂಡಾಗ ಅದು ನನಗೆ ನೋವು ಉಂಟಾಗುತ್ತದೆ.
    . ಹೌದು, ಬಿಟ್ಟು ಬಿಟ್ಟು
    . ಕೆಲವ್ಪೊಮ್ಮೆ
    . ಯಾವಾಗಲು ಇಲ್ಲ
    . ಇಲ್ಲವೇ ಇಲ್ಲ.

Khmer/Cambodian

តើអ្នកមានអារម្មណ៍យ៉ាងណាដែរ?

ដោយសារអ្នកទើបនឹងសំរាលកូនរួច សូមអ្នករៀបរាប់អំពីអារម្មណ៍របស់អ្នកក្នុងពេលឥឡូវនេះ។ សូមអ្នកគូសពីក្រោមចម្លើយណាមួយដែលត្រូវនឹងអារម្មណ៍របស់អ្នក ក្នុងកំឡុងពេលៗថ្ងៃកន្លងមកនេះ គឺមិនត្រឹមតែនៅថ្ងៃនេះទេ។ ខាងក្រោមនេះជាឧទាហរណ៍មួយដែលគេបំពេញរួចហើយ។ ខ្ញុំមានអារម្មណ៍សប្បាយរីករាយ:

ចាស ស្ទើរតែរាល់ពេល

<u>ចាស នៅពេលខ្លះៗ</u>

ទេ មិនសូវៃទេ

ទេ អត់ទាល់តែសោះ

ចម្លើយនេះបានសេចក្តីថា ខ្ញុំមានអារម្មណ៍សប្បាយរីករាយនៅពេលខ្លះក្នុងកំឡុងពេលៗថ្ងៃកន្លងមកនេះ។ សូមបំពេញសំនួរដទៃៗតាមរបៀបនេះ។

ក្នុងរយ:ពេលៗថ្ងៃកន្លងមកនេះ

១ - ខ្ញុំអាចលេងសើចបាន

ដូចធម្មតា

មិនសូវៃដូចពីមុនទេ

ប្រាកដជាមិនដូចពីមុនទេ

រកសើចមិនកើតទាល់តែសោះ

២ - ខ្ញុំចង់បានការសប្បាយរីករាយអំពីអ្វីៗ

ដូចចិត្តដែលធ្លាប់ចង់បានពីមុន

មិនសូវៃបានដូចពីមុនទេ

ប្រាកដជាមិនបានដូចពីមុនទេ

សឹងតែគ្មានចិត្តចង់ទាល់តែសោះ

៣ - ខ្ញុំបានផ្តោលទោសខ្លួនឯងពេលណាមានអ្វីខុស

ចាស ជារឿយៗ

ចាស ពេលខ្លះ

មិនញ៉ឹកញាប់ណាស់ទេ

ទេ មិនដែលសោះ

៤ - ខ្ញុំបានខ្វល់ខ្វាយឬព្រួយបារម្ភដោយមិនសមហេតុផល

ទេ អត់ទាល់តែសោះ

សឹងតែគ្មានសោះ

ចាស ជួនកាល

ចាស ញ៉ឹកញាប់ណាស់

(សូមឆ្លើយទៅនឹងសំនួរទី៥ទៅទី១០នៅទំព័រម្ខាងទៀតនេះ)

៥- ខ្ញុំបានភ័យខ្លាចឬស្ទើស្លោដោយមិនសមហេតុផល
    ចាស ញឹកញាប់ណាស់
    ចាស ជួនកាល
    ទេ មិនសូវទេ
    ទេ អត់ទាល់តែសោះ

៦- ខ្ញុំបានគ្រវីបញ្ហាជឿះជាន់ច្រើនហួស
    ចាស ខ្ញុំច្រើនតែមិនអាចទប់ទល់បានសោះ
    ចាស ជួនកាលខ្ញុំមិនអាចទប់ទល់បានដូចធម្មតាទេ
    ទេ ខ្ញុំតែងតែទប់ទល់បានល្អដែរ
    ទេ ខ្ញុំអាចទប់ទាល់បានដូចធម្មតា

៧- ខ្ញុំបានព្រួយចិត្តពេកទាល់តែដេកមិនបាន
    ចាស ស៊ីងតែគ្រប់ពេល
    ចាស ញឹកញាប់ណាស់ដែរ
    ទេ មិនសូវទេ
    ទេ អត់ទាល់តែសោះ

៨- ខ្ញុំបានមានការព្រួយឬវេទនាចិត្ត
    ចាស គ្រប់ពេលវេលា
    ចាស ញឹកញាប់ណាស់ដែរ
    ទេ មិនសូវទេ
    ទេ អត់ទាល់តែសោះ

៩- ខ្ញុំបានព្រួយចិត្តពេកទាល់តែយំ
    ចាស ស៊ីងតែគ្រប់ពេលវេលា
    ចាស ញឹកញាប់ណាស់ដែរ
    ម្ដងម្កាលប៉ុណ្ណោះ
    ទេ អត់ទាល់តែសោះ

១០- ខ្ញុំបានមានអារម្មណ៍ចង់ធ្វើអំពើហ៊ង្សាដល់ខ្លួនឯង
    ចាស ញឹកញាប់ណាស់
    ជួនកាល
    ស៊ីងតែគ្មានសោះ
    មិនដែលសោះឡើយ

© The Royal College of Psychiatrists 1987.

Konkani

1. Jednam kasli mhajechi ghosht gadta tedna tu hasunk shakta?
   I have been able to laugh and see the funny side of things

0	a. Soddanche baxen *As much as I always could*
1	b. Atam titlemxem nam *Not quite so much now*
2	c. Atam xert title nam *Definitely not so much now*
3	d. Samkench na *Not at all*

2. Tu fudarakaden ummedin paraita?
   I have looked forward with enjoyment to things.

0	a. Poilibashen *As much as I ever did*
1	b. Poiliparas matxe kami *Rather less than I used to*
2	c. Poiliparas samkench kami *Definitely less than I used to*
3	d. Chadxem nanch *Hardly at all*

3. Kenna vait zalear tu karan nastana tuka doshi tharaita?
   I have blamed myself unnecessarily when things went wrong.

3	a. Hai, khubhxe paut *Yes, most of the time*
2	b. Hai , Kenna-kenna *Yes , some of the time*
1	c. Chodxem na *Not very often*
0	d. Na, kennach na *No, never*

4. Kaench karan nastana tu chintest vo nervous zalea?
   I have felt worried and anxious for no very good reason.

0	a. Na, kennach na *No, not at all*
1	b. Chodxem na *Hardly ever*
2	c. Hai, kennai *Yes, sometimes*
3	d. Hai, jaite pauti *Yes, very often*

5. Kaench karan nastana tu beili ani tujer akanth ailo?
   I have felt scared and panicky for no good reason.

3	a. Hai , khub pauti *Yes, quite a lot*
2	b. Hai, kenna-kenna *Yes, sometimes*
1	c. Chodxem na *No, not much*
0	d. Na, kennach na *No, not at all*

6. Sogle ghazalincho tujer pez eila oxem uka dista?
   Things have been getting on top of me.

3	a. Hai, Soddanch *Yes, most of the time I haven't been able to cope at all*
2	b. Hai, kenna-kenna *Yes, sometimes I haven't been coping as well as usual*
1	c. Na, chodd na *No, most of the time I have been coping quite well*
0	d. Na, kainch na *No, I have been coping as well as usual*

7. Tu itli dukhi asta ki tuka nidh podona?
   I have been so unhappy I have had difficulty sleeping.
   - 3   a. Hai, khub pauti *Yes, most of the time*
   - 2   b. Hai, kenna-kenna *Yes, some of the time*
   - 1   c. Chadxe na *Not very often*
   - 0   d. Na, kennach na *No, not at all*

8. Tu dukhest/udhas va mhon padillea baxen zalli?
   I have felt sad or miserable.
   - 3   a. Hai, khubshe pauti *Yes, most of the time*
   - 2   b. Hai, kenna-kenna *Yes, quite often*
   - 1   c. Chodshe na *Not very often*
   - 0   d. Na, kennach na *No, not at all*

9. Tu, itli dukhi asta ki tu radta?
   I have been so unhappy that I have been crying.
   - 3   a. Hai, khub paut *Yes, most of the time*
   - 2   b. Hai, chodxe *Yes, some of the time*
   - 1   c. Kennai *Not very often*
   - 0   d. Na, kennach na *No not at all*

10. Jivache vait karpache vichar tujea mhonnat eitat?
    The thought of harming myself has occurred to me.
    - 3   a. Hai, khub pauti *Yes, quite often*
    - 2   b. Kenna-kenna *Sometimes*
    - 1   c. Chodxe na *Hardly ever*
    - 0   d. Kennach na *Never*

Korean

곧 출산을 앞두고 계시거나, 최근 출산을 하신 분들을 대상으로 심리상태를 알아보고자
합니다.오늘의 심리상태가 아니라 최근 7일동안 귀하께서 느끼신 감정에 가장 가까운 답변에
체크해 주시기 바랍니다.

이미 작성된 아래의 예를 참조하시기 바랍니다:

저는 최근 행복하다고 느꼈습니다:
[ ] 예, 항상 그러하였습니다.
[x] 예, 대부분의 경우 (대체로) 그러하였습니다.
[ ] 아니오, 별로 그렇지 않았습니다.
[ ] 아니오, 전혀 그렇지 않았습니다.

예문의 경우: 답변자가 지난 1주일 동안 "대부분의 경우 (대체로) 행복하다고 느꼈다'고 대답을
한 것입니다. 예문과 마찬가지로 다음의 질문들에 답변해 주시기 바랍니다.

지난 7 일 동안:

1. 나는 잘 웃고 주변 일들의 재미난 면을 잘 볼 수 있었습니다.
[ ] 예전과 마찬가지로 그러하였습니다.
[ ] 예전보다는 조금 덜 그러하였습니다.
[ ] 예전보다 확실히 많이 그러하지 못하였습니다.
[ ] 전혀 그렇지 못하였습니다.

2. 나는 즐거운 마음으로 미래에 일어날 일들을 기대하였습니다.
[ ] 예전과 마찬가지로 그러하였습니다.
[ ] 예전보다는 조금 덜 그러하였습니다.
[ ] 예전보다는 확실히 덜 그러하였습니다.
[ ] 거의 그러하지 못하였습니다.

3. 일이 잘못될 경우 나는 지나치게 나 스스로를 탓하였습니다.
[ ] 예, 대부분의 경우 (대체로) 그러하였습니다.
[ ] 예, 종종 그러하였습니다.
[ ] 자주 그렇지는 않았습니다.
[ ] 아니요, 전혀 그렇지 않았습니다.

4. 나는 특별한 이유 없이 초조하고 불안하였습니다.
[ ] 아니요, 전혀 그렇지 않았습니다.
[ ] 거의 그렇지 않았습니다.
[ ] 예, 때때로 그러하였습니다.
[ ] 예, 자주 그러하였습니다.

5. 나는 뚜렷한 이유 없이 두려움 혹은 공포심을 느꼈습니다.
[ ] 예, 꽤 자주 그러하였습니다.
[ ] 예, 종종 그러하였습니다.
[ ] 아니요, 그다지 그렇지 않았습니다.
[ ] 아니요, 전혀 그렇지 않았습니다.

6. 상황이 내게는 너무 버겁게 느껴졌습니다.
[ ] 예, 대부분의 경우 상황을 전혀 감당할 수 없었습니다.
[ ] 예, 예전처럼 상황을 처리하지 못하는 때가 종종 있었습니다.
[ ] 아니요, 대부분의 경우 상황을 잘 처리할 수 있었습니다.
[ ] 아니요, 늘 그렇듯이 상황을 잘 처리했습니다.

7. 나는 너무 불행해서 잠을 이루기가 어려웠습니다.
[ ] 예, 대부분의 경우 그러하였습니다.
[ ] 예, 종종 그러하였습니다.
[ ] 아니요, 자주 그렇지는 않았습니다.
[ ] 아니요, 전혀 그렇지 않았습니다.

8. 나는 슬프고 비참하다고 느꼈습니다.
[ ] 예, 대부분의 경우 그러하였습니다.
[ ] 예, 꽤 자주 그러하였습니다.
[ ] 아니요, 자주 그렇지는 않았습니다.
[ ] 아니요, 전혀 그렇지 않았습니다.

9. 너무 불행하다고 느껴서 울었습니다.
[ ] 예, 대부분의 경우 그러하였습니다.
[ ] 예, 꽤 자주 그러하였습니다.
[ ] 아주 가끔 그러하였습니다.
[ ] 아니요, 전혀 그렇지 않았습니다.

10. 자해하고 싶다는 생각이 들었습니다.
[ ] 예, 꽤 자주 그러하였습니다.
[ ] 때때로 그러하였습니다.
[ ] 거의 그렇지 않았습니다.
[ ] 전혀 그렇지 않았습니다.

Kurdish

لیستی‌نیشان : پێوەری ئەدنبر بۆخەمۆکی دوای مندالبوون

1- توانیومه پێبکەنم و لایەنی سەیرو خۆش و جوانەکانی شتان ببینم.

0- ئەوەندەی له توانامدابوو بێت.

1- ئێستا وا زۆر نا

2- به دڵنیایەوە ئێستا زۆر نه

3- به هیچ شێوەیەك نەمتوانیه

2- به خۆشیەوە تەماشای پێشەوە م کردووه و چێژم وەرگرتووه له شتەکان

0- وەك جاران

1- تۆزێ کەمتر له جاران

2- به مسۆگەری کەمتر له جاران

3-به زەحمەت (هەرگیز)

3- به شێوەیەکی نا پێویست سەرزەنشتی خۆم کردووه، کاتێك شتەکان به پێچەوانەی خواستی خۆم بوون.

3- بەلێ زۆربەی کات

2- بەلێ هەندێ جار

1- زۆر نا

0- نا، هەرگیز

4- دڵه راوکێم هەبووه یان نیگەران بوومه به بێ هۆی گونجاو

0- نەخێر هیچ جارێك

1- به زەحمەت (به کەمی)

2- بەلێ هێندی جار

3- بەلێ زۆر جار

5- هەست به ترسم کردووه یان زراوم چووه به هیچ هۆیەکی گونجاو

3- بەلێ زۆر جار

2- بەلێ هەندێ جار

1- نەخێر زۆر نا

0- نەخێر ، هیچ کاتێك

6- شتەکان له سەرم کۆ بوونەوەدو کەلەکه دەبوون.

3- بەلێ زۆربەی جار نەمتوانیوه خۆم بگونجینم

2- بەلێ هەندێك جار نەمتوانیوه وەك پێویست خۆم بگۆنجینم

1- نەخێر زۆربەی جار باش گۆنجاوم

0- نەخێر باش گۆنجاوم وەك جاران

7- ئەوەندە غەمبار و دڵتەند بوومە کە خەوم لێ تێکچووە.

3- بەڵێ زۆربەی جار

2- بەڵێ هەندێ جار

1- زۆر نا

0- نەخێر هیچ کاتێك

8- هەستم بە خەفەتباری یان شپرزەیی کردووە.

3- بەڵێ زۆربەی کات

2- بەڵێ هەندێك جار

1- زۆر نا

0- نەخێر هیچ کاتێك

9- ئەوەندە غەمبار بووم لە ئەنجامدا گریاوم.

3- بەڵێ زۆربەی کات

2- بەڵێ هەندێك جار

1- جار جار

0- نەخێر هەرگیز

10- بیری خۆ ئازاردانم بۆ هاتووە.

3- بەڵێ زۆربەی کات

2- بەڵێ هەندێك جار

1- زۆر بە دەگمەن

0- نەخێر هەرگیز

Lithuanian

Gerbiama ponia,
Mes norėtume sužinoti, kaip Jūs jaučiatės. <u>PABRAUKITE</u> atsakymą, kuris artimiausias Jūsų savijautai per pastarąsias SEPTYNIAS DIENAS (neapsiribokite savijauta šiandien). Čia pateikiamas pavyzdys kaip reikia pildyti:

Aš jaučiausi linksma:
<u>Taip, visa laiką</u>
Taip, didžiąją laiko dalį
Ne, nelabai dažnai
Ne, visiškai ne

1. Aš galėjau juoktis ir matyti linksmas gyvenimo puses:
   Taip kaip visada
   Dabar kiek mažiau
   Dabar žymiai mažiau
   Visiškai ne

2. Aš žvelgiau į ateitį su džiaugsmu:
   Taip kaip visada
   Kiek mažiau nei anksčiau
   Žymiai mažiau nei anksčiau
   Visiškai ne

3. Aš be reikalo kaltindavau save, jeigu nepasisekdavo:
   Dažniausiai
   Kartais
   Retai
   Niekada

4. Aš jausdavausi be priežasties nerami ir susirūpinusi:
   Visiškai ne
   Labai retai
   Kartais
   Labai dažnai

5. Aš be rimtos priežasties jausdavausi išsigandusi ar apimta panikos:
   Gana dažnai
   Kartais
   Neypatingai
   Visiškai ne

6. Aš negaliu išspręsti kylančių problemų:
   Taip, didžiąją laiko dalį aš visiškai nepajėgiu jų išspręsti
   Taip, kartais aš nepajėgiu iššspręsti taip sėkmingai kaip anksčiau
   Ne, didžiąją laiko dalį aš susitvarkau
   Ne, aš susitvarkau kaip visada

7. Aš tokia nelaiminga, kad pradėjau blogai miegoti:
   Taip, didžiąją laiko dalį
   Gana dažnai
   Kartais
   Visiškai ne

8. Aš jaučiausi liūdna ar suvargusi:
   Taip, didžiąją laiko dalį
   Taip, gana dažnai
   Kartais
   Visiškai ne

9. Aš tokia nelaiminga, kad net verkdavau:
   Taip, didžiąją laiko dalį
   Gana dažnai
   Tik kartais
   Niekada

10. Man kildavo mintys susižaloti:
    Gana dažnai
    Kartais
    Labai retai
    Niekada

Macedonian

Како се чувствувате?
Доколку неодамна имавте бебе, ние би сакале да знаеме како сега се чувствувате. Ве молиме подвлечете го одговорот што е најблизу до она како се чувствувавте во изминативе 7 дена, а не само како се чувствувате денеска. Еве еден пополнет пример:

Се чувствував среќно:
    Да, најголемиот дел од времето
    <u>Да, за извесно време</u>
    Не, не многу
    Не, воопшто не

Ова би значело: 'Се чувствував среќно за извесно време во текот на изминатата недела.'

Ве молиме одговорете ги останатите прашања на истиот начин.

Во изминатите 7 дена

1. Бев во состојба да се смеам и да ја согледам смешната страна на работите:
    Толку колку и секогаш
    Сега не толку многу
    Не, дефинитивно не толку многу
    Воопшто не

2. Со задоволство бев во исчекување на нешта:
    Така како што сум секогаш
    Многу помалку отколку порано
    Дефинитивно помалку отколку порано
    Речиси воопшто не

3. Се обвинував себеси кога работите одеа во погрешен правец:
    Да, најголемиот дел од времето
    Да, за извесно време
    Не многу често
    Не, никогаш

4. Бев нервозна или загрижена без некоја добра причина:
    Не, воопшто не
    Речиси никогаш
    Да, понекогаш
    Да, многу често

5. Се чувствував уплашено или воспаничено без некоја добра причина:
   Да, доста често
   Да, понекогаш
   Не, не многу
   Не, воопшто не

6. Работите ми претставуваа преоптоварување:
   Да, најголемиот дел од времето не бев во состојба да издржам
   Да, понекогаш не бев толку издржлива како нормално
   Не, најголем дел од времето издржував прилично добро
   Не, издржував добро како и секогаш

7. Бев толку несреќна што имав потешкотии со спиењето:
   Да, најголемиот дел од времето
   Да, доста често
   Не многу често
   Не, никогаш

8. Се чувствував тажно или мизерно:
   Да, најголемиот дел од времето
   Да, доста често
   Не многу често
   Не, воопшто не

9. Бев толку несреќна што плачев:
   Да, најголемиот дел од времето
   Да, доста често
   Само понекогаш
   Не, никогаш

10. Ми доаѓаа мисли да се повредам себеси:
    Да, доста често
    Понекогаш
    Скоро никогаш
    Никогаш

Malay

Kami ingin mengetahui perasaan dan keadaan anda pada 7 hari kebelakangan ini. Sila tandakan jawapan yang paling tepat menggambarkan keadaan diri anda.

Contohnya: Saya merasa gembira
a) Sentiasa [ ]
b) Kadangkala [/]
c) Kebanyakan waktu [ ]
d) Jarang sekali [ ]

Nota: Sila tandakan [/] di dalam ruang yang disediakan.

Ini bermaksud 'Saya merasa gembira <u>kadangkala</u> sepanjang minggu ini'. Sila tandakan jawapan seterusnya dengan cara yang sama.

Dalam masa 7 hari yang lalu

1. Saya berupaya untuk ketawa dan melihat kelucuan sesuatu perkara itu
   0 Sebanyak mungkin seperti biasa [ ]
   1 Kurang daripada biasa [ ]
   2 Jarang sekali pada masa ini [ ]
   3 Tiada langsung [ ]

2. Saya telah dapat melihat kehadapan dengan perasaan gembira terhadap perkara-perkara yang bakal berlaku.
   0 Sebanyak mungkin seperti biasanya [ ]
   1 Kurang dari yang pernah saya biasa buat [ ]
   2 Jarang sekali pada masa ini [ ]
   3 Tidak pernah langsung [ ]

3. Saya telah menyalahkan diri sendiri secara tidak sepatutnya apabila terjadi sesuatu yang buruk
   3 Ya, kebanyakannya [ ]
   2 Ya, kadangkala [ ]
   1 Tidak, jarang sekali [ ]
   0 Tidak, tidak pernah [ ]

4. Saya telah merasa bimbang dan rungsing tanpa sebab-sebab yang munasabah
   0 Tidak, tidak pernah [ ]
   1 Ya, jarang sekali [ ]
   2 Ya, kadang-kadang [ ]
   3 Ya, seringkali [ ]

5. Saya telah merasa takut ataupun gugup tanpa sebab yang munasabah
   - 3 Ya, kerapkali [ ]
   - 2 Ya, kadangkala [ ]
   - 1 Tidak, jarang sekali [ ]
   - 0 Tidak, tidak pernah [ ]

6. Perkara-perkara yang telah membebankan fikiran saya
   - 3 Ya, kebanyakan masa saya sama sekali tidak dapat mengatasinya [ ]
   - 2 Ya, kadang-kala saya tidak dapat mengatasinya sebaik biasa [ ]
   - 1 Tidak, kebanyakan masa saya mampu mengatasinya sebaik mungkin [ ]
   - 0 Tidak, saya telah dapat mengatasinya sebaik mungkin [ ]

7. Saya telah merasa sungguh sedih sehingga saya mengalami kesukaran untuk tidur
   - 3 Ya, kebanyakan masa [ ]
   - 2 Ya, kadang-kala [ ]
   - 1 Tidak , jarang sekali [ ]
   - 0 Tidak, tidak pernah [ ]

8. Saya telah merasa sedih atau dukacita
   - 3 Ya, kebanyakan masa [ ]
   - 2 Ya, agak kerap [ ]
   - 1 Tidak berapa kerap [ ]
   - 0 Tidak, tidak pernah [ ]

9. Saya telah merasa begitu sedih sehingga saya menangis
   - 3 Ya, kebanyakan masa [ ]
   - 2 Ya, agak kerap [ ]
   - 1 Cuma sekali sekala [ ]
   - 0 Tidak, tidak pernah [ ]

10. Perasaan untuk mencederakan diri sendiri pernah terlintas di fikiran saya
    - 3 Ya, kebanyakan masa [ ]
    - 2 Ya, agak kerap [ ]
    - 1 Cuma sekala sekali [ ]
    - 0 Tidak pernah terlintas [ ]

Maltese

Kif qed thossok?

Wara t-twelid tat-tarbija tiegħek, nixtiequ nkunu nafu kif qed thossok. Jekk jogħġbok immarka risposta waħda li thoss li tgħodd fil-kas tiegħek, ta' kif hassejtek f'dawn l-aħħar sebat ijiem, u mhux kif qed thossok illum. Hawn taħt hawn eżempju diġà lest.

> Jiena hassejtni ferħana:
>> Iva, il-hin kollu
>> <u>Iva, hafna drabi</u>
>> Le, mhux ta' spiss
>> Le, qatt
> Din tkun tfisser li "jien hassejtni ferħana hafna drabi" f'din l-aħħar ġimgħa.

Jekk jogħġbok immarka r-risposti l-oħrajn bl-istess mod.

FL-AĦĦAR SEBAT IJIEM

1. Kont kapaċi nifraħ u nhares lejn is-sabiħ tal-ħajja:
     Bhas-soltu
     Mhux daqs is-soltu
     Żgur li mhux bhas-soltu
     Żgur li le

2. Kien ikolli ċertu heġġa għal dak li nkun ser nagħmel:
     Bhas-soltu
     Aktarx inqas mis-soltu
     Żgur li inqas mis-soltu
     Ftit li xejn

3. Tajt tort lili nnifsi għal xejn b'xejn meta l-affarijiet marru ħazin:
     Kwazi dejjem
     Iva, kulltant
     Mhux ta'spiss
     Le, qatt

4. Hassejtni nervuża u nkwietata għal xejn b'xejn:
     Le, lanqas xejn
     Rari ħafna
     Iva, kulltant
     Iva, ta' spiss

5. Hassejtni beżgħana u qabadni paniku anke għal xejn b'xejn
     Iva, hafna drabi
     Iva, kulltant
     Le, mhux ta' spiss
     Le, qatt

6. Ma stajt inlaħħaq ma xejn
     Iva, hafna drabi hassejtni li ma stajtx inlaħħaq
     Iva, kulltant hassejtni li ma kontx kapaċi nlaħħaq bhas-soltu
     Le, hafna drabi stajt nlaħħaq
     Le, laħħaqt bhas-soltu

7. Tant ħassejtni mdejqa li kont insibha bi tqila biex norqod
>Kważi dejjem
>Iva, kulltant
>Mhux ta' spiss
>Le, qatt

8. Ħassejtni mdejqa u miżerabbli
>Iva, kważi l-ħin kollu
>Iva ta' spiss
>Le, mhux ta' spiss
>Le, qatt

9. Tant ħassejtni mdejqa li kulltant kien itini l-biki
>Iva, kważi l-ħin kollu
>Iva, ta' spiss
>Xi kulltant
>Le, qatt

10. Kienu jiġuni xi ħsibijiet li nagħmel ħsara lili nnifsi
>Iva, ta' spiss
>Xi, kulltant
>Rari, ħafna
>Qatt

Myanmar/Burmese

စိတ်ထဲဘယ်လိုရှိနေလဲ?

မကြာခင်ကဘဲ ကလေးမွေးခဲ့တာမို့၊ အခုစိတ်ထဲ ဘယ်လိုခံစားနေရလဲ ဆိုတာသိလိုပါတယ်။ ဒီနေ့မှာ ခံစားနေရတာ သက်သက်မဟုတ်ဘဲ၊ ပြီးခဲ့တဲ့ (၇)ရက်အတွင်း ခံစားခဲ့ရတာနဲ့ အနီးစပ်ဆုံးအဖြေကို အောက်မျဉ်းတားပေးပါ။ ဥပမာအားဖြင့် အဖြေပေးထားတာ တစ်ခုပြရမယ် ဆိုရင်–

ကျွန်မ ပျော်ပျော်ရွှင်ရွှင် စိတ်ရှိခဲ့ပါတယ် –

ဟုတ်ကဲ့၊ အမြဲတမ်းလိုလိုပါဘဲ
ဟုတ်ကဲ့၊ တခါတရံပါဘဲ
သိပ်မရှိလှဘူး
လုံးဝမပျော်ပါဘူး

ဆိုလိုတာက– "ပြီးခဲ့တဲ့ တစ်ပါတ်အတွင်း ပျော်ရွှင်တဲ့စိတ် တခါတရံ ရှိခဲ့ပါတယ်။"

အောက်ပါမေးခွန်းများကို ယင်းကဲ့သို့ ဖြေပေးပါ။

ပြီးခဲ့တဲ့(၇)ရက်အတွင်း

၁။ ရီမောစရာများရှိခဲ့ရင်၊ ရီနိုင်ခဲ့တယ် –

အရင်ကအတိုင်း ရီမောနိုင်ပါတယ်။
အခု အရင်ကလောက် မရီနိုင်တော့ဘူး။
သေချာပေါက် အရင်ကလောက် မရီနိုင်တော့ဘူး။
လုံးဝ မရီနိုင်တော့ဘူး။

၂။ ပျော်ရွှင်စရာများ လုပ်ဆောင်ရန်၊ မျှော်လင့်နေတတ်တယ် –

အရင်က ပုံစံအတိုင်းဘဲ
အရင်ကထက်တော့ နည်းသွားတယ်။
အရင်ကထက် သေချာပေါက် နည်းသွားပြီ။
မရှိသလောက်ဘဲ။

၃။ အဆင်မပြေ ဖြစ်သွားတာတွေအတွက်၊ ကိုယ့်ကိုကိုယ် အပြစ်တင်မိတယ် –

ဟုတ်ကဲ့၊ အမြဲလိုလိုဘဲ။
ဟုတ်ကဲ့၊ တခါတရံပါဘဲ။
လုပ်ခဲပါတယ်။
တစ်ခါမှ မဖြစ်ပါဘူး။

၄။ အကြောင်းမရှိဘဲ၊ ပူပန်စိုးရိမ်နေမိတယ် –

လုံးဝမဖြစ်ပါဘူး။
မဖြစ်သလောက်ပါဘဲ။
တခါတလေပါဘဲ။
တော်တော်များများဖြစ်ပါတယ်။ (တဖက်မှ မေးခွန်း ၅–၁၀ ကိုဖြေပါ)

၅။ လုံလောက်တဲ့ အကြောင်းမရှိဘဲ၊ ကြောက်လန့်တုန်လှုပ်စိတ်တွေ ဖြစ်နေမိတယ် –

တော်တော်များများဘဲ။
တခါတရံ ဖြစ်ပါတယ်။
သိပ်မဖြစ်ပါဘူး။
လုံးဝမဖြစ်ပါဘူး။

၆။ ဘာဘဲလုပ်လုပ် မပြီးစီးနိုင်ဘူး –

ဟုတ်ကဲ့၊ မနိုင်မနင်းဖြစ်တဲ့စိတ် အတော်များနေပါတယ်။
ဟုတ်ကဲ့၊ အရင်တုန်းကလိုမျိုး နိုင်နိုင်နင်းနင်း မရှိလှဘူး။
များသောအားဖြင့် နိုင်နိုင်နင်းနင်း ရှိပါတယ်။
အရင်အတိုင်း နိုင်နိုင်နင်းနင်းပါဘဲ။

၇။ ကျွန်မမှာ စိတ်မချမ်းမသာဖြစ်လွန်းလို့၊ ကောင်းကောင်းအိပ်လို့မရခဲ့ဘူး –
      ဟုတ်ကဲ့၊ အမြဲလိုလိုဘဲ။
      ဟုတ်ကဲ့၊ မကြာခဏဘဲ။
      သိပ်မဖြစ်လှဘူး။
      လုံးဝမဖြစ်ပါဘူး။

၈။ ဝမ်းနည်း/စိတ်ဆင်းရဲဖြစ်နေခဲ့တယ် –
      အမြဲလိုလိုဘဲ။
      မကြာခဏဘဲ။
      သိပ်မဖြစ်လှဘူး။
      လုံးဝမဖြစ်ပါဘူး။

၉။ ကျွန်မမှာ စိတ်မချမ်းမသာဖြစ်လွန်းလို့ ငိုနေမိတယ်–
      အမြဲလိုလိုဘဲ။
      မကြာခဏဘဲ။
      သိပ်မဖြစ်လှဘူး။
      လုံးဝမဖြစ်ပါဘူး။

၁၀။ ကိုယ့်ကိုကိုယ် အန္တရာယ်ပြုဖို့ စိတ်ကူးမိခဲ့တယ် –
      ဟုတ်ကဲ့၊ မကြာခဏဘဲ။
      တခါတရံ။
      မဖြစ်သလောက်ဘဲ။
      လုံးဝမဖြစ်ပါ။

Nepali

निर्देशन

तपाईंको हालसालै बच्चा भएकाले तपाईंलाई अहिले कस्तो छ, त्यो हामी जान्न चाहन्छौं । तपाई गत हप्ता, (अहिले जस्तो मात्र हैन), कस्तो हुनु हुन्थ्यो ? तल दिएका उत्तरहरु मध्ये नबेभन्दा मिल्दो उत्तरमा चिन्हो लगाउनुहोस् ।

मिति

गतहप्तामा

१. मैले जीवनका रमाइला क्षणहरुलाई बुभ्रन र त्यसमाथि हास्न सकें
– आफूले बुभ्रन र हास्न सकें
– अहिले त्यति गर्न सकिन
– पक्कै त्यति गर्न सकिन
– कहिल्यै पनि बुभ्रन र हास्न सकिन

२. मैले आशावादी भएर भविष्यलाई हेरें ।
– पहिले कहिल्यै पनि नहेरें भैं
– पहिले भन्दा अलि कम
– पहिले भन्दा पक्कै कम
– कहिल्यै पनि हेरिन

३. काम विग्रेमा मैले आफुलाई अनावश्यक रुपले दोषी ठहऱ्याएं ।
– अ, धेरै जसो
– अ, कहिलेकांही
– कुनै वेला मात्र
– कहिल्यै पनि दोषी ठहराइन

४. बिना कारण म चिन्तित भइरहेको छु
– कहिल्यै पनि भएको छैन
– धेरै नै कम
– अ, कहिलेकांही
– अ, प्राय: जसो

५. बिना कारण म डराएं वा आत्तिएं
– अ, प्राय: धेरै जसो वेला
– अ, कहिलेकांही
– अहँ, त्यति डराइन
– अहँ, कहिल्यै पनि डराइन

६. म धेरै जसो भन्भटमा फंसेको छु
– अ, धेरै जसो भन्भटबाट मुक्त हुन सकिन
– अ, कहिलेकांही म भन्भटबाट मुक्त हुन सकिन
– प्राय जसो म भन्भटबाट मुक्त हुन सकें
– हो, सधैं भैं म भन्भटबाट मुक्त हुन सकें

७. म यति दु:खी छु कि मलाई निद्रा लाग्दैन
– अ, धेरै जसो
– अ, कहिलेकांही
– कुनै वेला मात्र
– कहिल्यै पनि लाग्दैन

८. मलाई विरक्त लागेको छ
– अ, धेरै जसो वेला
– अ, प्राय: जसो
– कहिलकांही मात्र
– कहिल्यै पनि लागेको छैन

९. म यति दु:खी छु कि जस कारण सधै रोइरहेको छु
– अ, धेरै जसो
– अ, प्राय: जसो
– कहिलेकांही मात्र
– होइन, कहिल्यै पनि रोएको छैन

१०. आफुलाई नोक्सान पार्ने विचार मनमा आएको छ ।
– अ, प्राय: जसो
– कहिलेकांही
– कुनै वेला मात्र
– कहिल्यै पनि आएन

पूर्ण प्राप्ताङ्क:

Norwegian

1. Har du siste 7 dager kunnet le og se det komiske i en situasjon?
   Like mye som vanlig
   Ikke riktig så mye som jeg pleier
   Klart mindre enn jeg pleier
   Ikke i det hele tatt

2. Har du siste 7 dager gledet deg til ting som skulle skje?
   Like mye som vanlig
   Noe mindre enn jeg pleier
   Klart mindre enn jeg pleier
   Nesten ikke i det hele tatt

3. Har du siste 7 dager bebreidet deg selv uten grunn når noe gikk galt?
   Ja, nesten hele tiden
   Ja, av og til
   Ikke saerlig ofte
   Nei aldri

4. Har du siste 7 dager vaert nerves eller bekymret uten grunn?
   Nei, slett ikke
   Nesten aldri
   Ja, iblant
   Ja, veldig ofte

5. Har du siste 7 dager vaert redd eller fått panikk uten grunn?
   Ja, svaert ofte
   Ja, noen ganger
   Sjelden
   Nei, aldri

6. Har du siste 7 dager folt at det har blitt for mye for deg?
   Ja, jeg har stort sett ikke fungert i det hele tatt
   Ja, iblant har jeg ikke klart å fungere som jeg pleier
   Nei, for det meste har jeg klart meg bra
   Nei, jeg har klart meg like bra som vanlig

7. Har du siste 7 dager vaert så ulykkelig at du har hatt vanskeligheter
   med å sove?
   Ja, for det meste
   Ja, iblant
   Ikke saerlig ofte
   Nei, ikke i det hele tatt

8. Har du siste 7 dager felt deg nedfor eller ulykkelig?
   Ja, det meste av tiden
   Ja, ganske ofte
   Ikke saerlig ofte
   Nei, ikke i det hele tatt

9. Har du siste 7 dager vaert så ulykkelig at du har grått?
   Ja, nesten hele tiden
   Ja, veldig ofte
   Ja, det har skjedd iblant
   Nei, aldri

10. Har tanken på å skade deg selv streifet deg, de siste 7 dagene?
    Ja, nokså ofte
    Ja, av og til
    Ja, såvidt
    Aldri

Polish

Proszę wybrać i podkreślić tę z odpowiedzi umieszczonych pod każdym z poniższych stwierdzeń, która najlepiej odpowiada temu, jak czuła się Pani w ciągu ostatnich siedmiu dni.

Proszę podkreślić tylko jedną odpowiedź w przypadku każdego zadania.

W ciągu ostatnich 7 dni:

1   Mogłam się śmiać i byłam zdolna zauważać zabawne strony tego, co się dzieje:
     tak samo, jak mogłam zawsze
     niezupełnie tak samo jak zawsze
     zdecydowanie nie tak samo jak zawsze
     wcale nie mogłam.

2   Z radością oczekiwałam tego, co nastąpi:
     tak samo, jak zawsze
     raczej z mniejszą radością niż zwykle
     ze zdecydowanie mniejszą radością
     wcale nie.

3   Gdy wydarzyło się coś złego uważałam, że to moja wina:
     tak, w zdecydowanej większości przypadków
     tak, dość często
     raczej rzadko
     nie, nigdy.

4   Byłam zdenerwowana lub zmartwiona bez uzasadnionych powodów:
     nie, nigdy
     raczej nie
     tak, czasami
     tak, bardzo często.

5   Bardzo się bałam bez uzasadnionych powodów:
     tak, bardzo często
     tak, czasami
     nie, niewiele
     nie, wcale.

6   Nie mogłam sobie z niczym poradzić:
     tak, przez większość czasu nie byłam w stanie dać sobie z niczym rady
     tak, czasami nie radziłam sobie tak dobrze jak zwykle
     nie, przez większość czasu radziłam sobie dość dobrze
     nie, radziłam sobie tak dobrze, jak zwykle.

7   Byłam tak nieszczęśliwa, że nie mogłam spać:
        tak, większość czasu
        tak, czasami
        tylko czasami
        nie, nigdy.

8   Byłam smutna lub czułam się przygnębiona:
        tak, większość czasu
        tak, czasami
        tylko czasami
        nie, nigdy.

9   Byłam tak nieszczęśliwa, że płakałam:
        tak, większość czasu
        tak, czasami
        tylko czasami
        nie, nigdy.

10   Myślałam, żeby zrobić sobie coś złego:
        tak, dość często
        czasami
        rzadko kiedy
        nigdy.

Translated by E. Bielawska-Batorowicz

Portuguese

Como teve recentemente um bebé, gostaríamos de saber como se sente. Por favor, sublinhe a resposta que melhor indique o modo como se sente desde há 7 dias e não apenas hoje.

Aqui está um exemplo:

> Senti-me feliz:
> > Sim, sempre
> > Sim, quase sempre
> > Não, poucas vezes
> > Não, nunca

Isto quereria dizer: 'Senti-me feliz quase sempre durante os últimos sete dias'. Por favor, complete as outras questões do mesmo modo.

Desde há 7 dias

1. Tenho sido capaz de me rir e ver o lado divertido das coisas:
    Tanto como dantes
    Menos do que antes
    Muito menos do que antes
    Nunca

2. Tenho tido esperança no futuro:
    Tanta como sempre tive
    Bastante menos do que costumava ter
    Muito menos do que costumava ter
    Quase nenhuma

3. Tenho-me culpado sem necessidade quando as coisas correm mal:
    Sim, a maioria das vezes
    Sim, algumas vezes
    Raramente
    Não, nunca

4. Tenho estado ansiosa ou preocupada sem motivo:
    Não, nunca
    Quase nunca
    Sim, por vezes
    Sim, muitas vezes

5. Tenho-me sentido com medo, ou muito assustada, sem grande motivo:
    Sim, muitas vezes
    Sim, por vezes
    Não, raramente
    Não, nunca

6. Tenho sentido que são coisas demais para mim:
    Sim, a maioria das vezes não tenho conseguido resolvê-las
    Sim, por vezes não tenho conseguido resolvê-las como dantes
    Não, a maioria das vezes resolvo-as facilmente
    Não, resolvo-as tão bem como dantes

7. Tenho-me sentido tão infeliz que durmo mal:
    Sim, quase sempre
    Sim, por vezes
    Raramente
    Não, nunca

8. Tenho-me sentido triste ou muito infeliz:
    Sim, quase sempre
    Sim, muitas vezes
    Raramente
    Não, nunca

9. Tenho-me sentido tão infeliz que choro:
    Sim, quase sempre
    Sim, muitas vezes
    Só às vezes
    Não, nunca

10. Tive ideias de fazer mal a mim mesma;
    Sim, muitas vezes
    Por vezes
    Muito raramente
    Nunca

Punjabi

Kujh din pahilan tuhada bachha paeda hoiaa hae aatae eh jananna chahudae han ke tuseen kis taran maehsoos karde ho. Pishlae ik haphtae ton jis yaran vee tuseen maehsoos kita cee oos barae mehar-bani karke dhhuck veen khanae vich nishan laga-dioo.

Eh ik aapdea layee namoona tiar kita hoiaa hae (e.g.)

> Maen khush rahee cee
>> Bahut vaar
>> <u>Kayee vaar</u>
>> Bahut vaar nahin
>> Bilkul nahin

Aaseen nishan swal de dujae hissea wich laeeyah hae.

Pishlae sat dina vich

1. Meree hasnae khadnae dee isha cee
   Pehilan jinee hee
   Agae nalon ghat
   Kadae kadae
   Bil-kul nahin

2. Maen dilhon khushee de nal cam karna chohundee cee
   Peilan wang hee
   Agae nalon kujh ghat
   Bil-kul agae nalon ghat
   Kadae vee nahin

3. Maen binan kisae karan aapnae aapda kasoor samajh-dee cee
   Bahut var
   Kayee var
   Bahut var nahin
   Bil-kul nahin

4. Maen bina kisae khash karan hee chinta phikar kardee cee
   Kadae vee nahin
   Bahut hee ghat
   Kadae kadae
   Bahut var

5. Maen bina kisae khash karan toen hee dar atae ghabrahat mahaesoos kardee cee
   Bahut var
   Kadee kadae
   Bahut var nahin
   Bil-kul nahin

6. Maen innee udas cee ke maen kisae tarah de tangee jan fikar valee gall sahar nahin sakdee cee
   Bahut var
   Kayee var
   Pehilan nalon kujh ghat
   Agae wang hee

7. Maenu gaman de dukh nal neend nahin aaundee cee
   Bahut var
   Kadae kadae
   Bahut var nahin
   Bil-kul nahin

8. Maen udas rahindee cee
   Bahut var
   Kayee var
   Bahut var nahin
   Bil-kul nahin

9. Maen innee udas cee kae maen rondee rahindee cee
   Bahut var
   Kayee var
   Kadae kadae
   Bil-kul nahin

10. Mera dil karda cee kae maen aapnae aap noon kujh kar lavan
    Buhat var
    Kadae kadae
    Bahut var nahin
    Bil-kul nahin

Punjabi script

ਕੁਝ ਦਿਨ ਪਹਿਲਾਂ ਤੁਹਾਡਾ ਬੱਚਾ ਪੈਦਾ ਹੋਇਆ ਹੈ ਅਤੇ ਇਹ ਜਾਣਨਾ ਚਾਹੁੰਦੇ ਹਾਂ ਕਿ ਤੁਸੀਂ ਕਿਸ ਤਰ੍ਹਾਂ ਮਹਿਸੂਸ ਕਰਦੇ ਹੋ। ਪਿਛਲੇ ਇਕ ਹਫ਼ਤੇ ਤੋਂ ਜਿਸ ਤਰ੍ਹਾਂ ਵੀ ਤੁਸੀਂ ਮਹਿਸੂਸ ਕੀਤਾ ਸੀ, ਉਸ ਬਾਰੇ ਮਿਹਰਬਾਨੀ ਕਰਕੇ ਢੁਕਵੇਂ ਖਾਨੇ ਵਿਚ ਨਿਸ਼ਾਨ ਲਗਾ ਦਿਓ।

ਇਹ ਆਪ ਦੇ ਲਈ ਇਕ ਨਮੂਨਾ ਤਿਆਰ ਕੀਤਾ ਹੋਇਆ ਹੈ (ਜਿਵੇਂ ਕਿ)
ਮੈਂ ਖ਼ੁਸ਼ ਰਹੀ ਸੀ:
- ☐ ਬਹੁਤ ਵਾਰ
- ☒ ਕਈ ਵਾਰ
- ☐ ਬਹੁਤ ਵਾਰ ਨਹੀਂ
- ☐ ਬਿਲਕੁਲ ਨਹੀਂ

ਅਸੀਂ ਨਿਸ਼ਾਨ ਸਵਾਲ ਦੇ ਦੂਜੇ ਖਾਨੇ ਵਿਚ ਲਗਾਇਆ ਹੈ।

ਪਿਛਲੇ ਸੱਤ ਦਿਨ ਵਿਚ:

1. ਮੇਰੀ ਹੱਸਣ ਦੀ ਕਦੀ ਨਹੀਂ ਇੱਛਾ ਸੀ
   - ☐ ਪਹਿਲਾਂ ਜਿੰਨੀ ਹੀ
   - ☐ ਅੱਗੇ ਨਾਲੋਂ ਘੱਟ
   - ☐ ਕਦੀ ਕਦਾਈਂ
   - ☐ ਬਿਲਕੁਲ ਨਹੀਂ

2. ਮੈਂ ਦਿਲੋਂ ਖ਼ੁਸ਼ੀ ਦੇ ਨਾਲ ਕੰਮ ਕਰਨਾ ਚਾਹੁੰਦੀ ਸੀ
   - ☐ ਪਹਿਲਾਂ ਵਾਂਗ ਹੀ
   - ☐ ਅੱਗੇ ਨਾਲੋਂ ਕੁਝ ਘੱਟ
   - ☐ ਬਿਲਕੁਲ ਅੱਗੇ ਨਾਲੋਂ ਘੱਟ
   - ☐ ਕਦੋਂ ਵੀ ਨਹੀਂ

3. ਮੈਂ ਬਿਨਾਂ ਕਿਸੇ ਕਾਰਨ ਆਪਣੇ ਆਪ ਦਾ ਕਸੂਰ ਸਮਝਦੀ ਸੀ
   - ☐ ਬਹੁਤ ਵਾਰ
   - ☐ ਕਈ ਵਾਰ
   - ☐ ਬਹੁਤ ਵਾਰ ਨਹੀਂ
   - ☐ ਬਿਲਕੁਲ ਨਹੀਂ

4. ਮੈਂ ਬਿਨਾਂ ਕਿਸੇ ਖ਼ਾਸ ਕਾਰਨ ਹੀ ਚਿੰਤਾ ਫਿਕਰ ਕਰਦੀ ਸੀ
   - ☐ ਕਦੀ ਵੀ ਨਹੀਂ
   - ☐ ਬਹੁਤ ਹੀ ਘੱਟ
   - ☐ ਕਦੀ ਕਦੀ
   - ☐ ਬਹੁਤ ਵਾਰ

5. ਮੈਂ ਬਿਨਾਂ ਕਿਸੇ ਖ਼ਾਸ ਕਾਰਨ ਤੋਂ ਹੀ ਡਰ ਅਤੇ ਘਬਰਾਹਟ ਮਹਿਸੂਸ ਕਰਦੀ ਸੀ
   - ☐ ਬਹੁਤ ਵਾਰ
   - ☐ ਕਦੀ ਕਦਾਈਂ
   - ☐ ਬਹੁਤ ਵਾਰ ਨਹੀਂ
   - ☐ ਬਿਲਕੁਲ ਨਹੀਂ

6. ਮੈਂ ਇੰਨੀ ਉਦਾਸ ਸੀ ਕਿ ਮੈਂ ਕਿਸੇ ਤਰ੍ਹਾਂ ਦੇ ਟੰਗੇ ਜਾਣ ਦੇ ਫਿਕਰ ਵਾਲੀ ਗੱਲ ਸਹਾਰ ਨਹੀਂ ਸਕਦੀ ਸੀ
   - ☐ ਬਹੁਤ ਵਾਰ
   - ☐ ਕਦੀ ਕਦਾਈਂ
   - ☐ ਪਹਿਲੇ ਨਾਲੋਂ ਕੁਝ ਘੱਟ
   - ☐ ਅੱਗੇ ਵਾਂਗ ਹੀ

7. ਮੈਨੂੰ ਗ਼ਮਾਂ ਦੇ ਦੁੱਖ ਨਾਲ ਨੀਂਦ ਨਹੀਂ ਆਉਂਦੀ ਸੀ
   - ☐ ਬਹੁਤ ਵਾਰ
   - ☐ ਕਦੀ ਕਦਾਈਂ
   - ☐ ਪਹਿਲਾ ਨਾਲੋਂ ਕੁਝ ਘੱਟ
   - ☐ ਬਿਲਕੁਲ ਨਹੀਂ

8. ਮੈਂ ਉਦਾਸ ਰਹਿੰਦੀ ਸੀ
   - ☐ ਬਹੁਤ ਵਾਰ
   - ☐ ਕਈ ਵਾਰ
   - ☐ ਬਹੁਤ ਵਾਰ ਨਹੀਂ
   - ☐ ਬਿਲਕੁਲ ਨਹੀਂ

9. ਮੈਂ ਇੰਨੀ ਉਦਾਸ ਸੀ ਕਿ ਮੈਂ ਰੋਂਦੀ ਰਹਿੰਦੀ ਸੀ
   - ☐ ਬਹੁਤ ਵਾਰ
   - ☐ ਕਈ ਵਾਰ
   - ☐ ਕਦੀ ਕਦਾਈਂ
   - ☐ ਬਿਲਕੁਲ ਨਹੀਂ

10. ਮੇਰਾ ਦਿਲ ਕਰਦਾ ਸੀ ਕਿ ਮੈਂ ਆਪਣੇ ਆਪ ਨੂੰ ਕੁਝ ਕਰ ਲਵਾਂ
    - ☐ ਬਹੁਤ ਵਾਰ
    - ☐ ਕਦੀ ਕਦਾਈਂ
    - ☐ ਬਹੁਤ ਵਾਰ ਨਹੀਂ
    - ☐ ਬਿਲਕੁਲ ਨਹੀਂ

Romanian

In ultimele 7 zile

1. Ati putut sa radeti si sa vedeti partea amuzanta a lucrurilor?
    Atat de mult cat ati putut intotdeauna
    Nu prea in aceasta perioada
    Aproape deloc in aceasta perioada
    Deloc

2. Ati asteptat cu bucurie ca unele lucruri sa se intample?
    Atat cat ati facut-o intotdeauna
    Mai degraba mai putin decat inainte
    Cu siguranta mai putin decat inainte
    Chiar deloc

3. V-ati invinovatit fara rost atunci cand lucrurile au mers prost?**
    Da, majoritatea timpului
    Da, o parte din timp
    Nu foarte des
    Nu, niciodata

4. Ati fost agitata sau ingrijorata fara vreun motiv intemeiat?
    Nu, deloc
    Aproape niciodata
    Da, cateodata
    Da, foarte des

5. V-ati simtit speriata sau panicata fara vreun motiv intemeiat?**
    Da, destul de des
    Da, cateodata
    Nu, nu foarte des
    Nu, deloc

6. Ati simtit ca va depasesc lucrurile in ultimul timp(va coplesesc)?**
    Da, majoritatea timpului nu ati putut face fata deloc
    Da, cateodata nu ati facut fata la fel de bine ca de obicei
    Nu, majoritatea timpului ati facut fata chiar bine
    Nu, ati facut fata la fel de bine ca intotdeauna

7. V-ati simtit atat de nefericita incat sa aveti probleme cu dormitul?**
    Da, majoritatea timpului
    Da, cateodata
    Nu foarte des
    Nu, deloc

8. V-ati simtit trista sau nefericita?**
   Da, majoritatea timpului
   Da, destul de des
   Nu foarte des
   Nu, deloc

9. V-ati simtit atat de nefericita incat sa plangeti?**
   Da, destul de des
   Cateodata
   Aproape niciodata
   Niciodata

10. V-ati gandit la a va face rau singura?**
    Da, destul de des
    Cateodata
    Aproape niciodata
    Niciodata

Russian

Поскольку у Вас недавно родился младенец, нас интересует ваше самочувствие. Пожалуйста, выберите ответ, который лучше всего отражает ваше самочувствие в течение ПОСЛЕДНИХ 7 ДНЕЙ, а не то, как Вы себя чувствуете сегодня.

Пример, ответа подготовленного заранее.

У чувствовала себя счастливой:

☐ Да, все время
☒ Да, большую часть времени
☐ Нет, не очень часто
☐ Нет, совсем никогда

Это означало бы: "Я чувствовала себя счастливой большую часть времени в течение последней недели"

Пожалуйста , ответте   на остальные   вопросы, следуя этому   примеру

В течение последних 7 дней:

1.   Я могла смеяться и замечать смешное вокруг себя
        ☐ Так же, как обычно
        ☐ Несколько меньше чем обычно
        ☐ Нет, гораздо меньше чем обычно
        ☐ Нет, совсем не могла

2.   Я ощущала радость думая о будущем
        ☐ Так же, как обычно
        ☐ Несколько меньше, чем обычно
        ☐ Значительно меньше, чем обычно
        ☐ Практически никогда

3.   Я корила себя понапрасну, когда дела шли не так, как надо
        ☐ Да, все время
        ☐ Да, иногда
        ☐ Нет, не так часто
        ☐ Нет, практически никогда

4.   Я беспокоилась понапрасну
        ☐ Нет, никогда
        ☐ Нет, почти никогда
        ☐ Да, иногда
        ☐ Да, очень часто

*5 . Меня охватывали беспричинный страх и паника
   ☐ Да, почти все время
   ☐ Да, иногда
   ☐ Нет, очень редко
   ☐ Нет, не так часто

*6. На меня слишком много всего навалилось
   ☐ Да, я почти ни с чем не справлялась
   ☐ Да, иногда я кое с чем не справлялась
   ☐ Нет, по большей части я со всем справлялась
   ☐ Нет, я сравлялась со всем, как обычно

*7. Мне было так плохо, что я не могла спать
   ☐ Да, почти каждую ночь
   ☐ Да, иногда
   ☐ Нет, очень редко
   ☐ Нет, не так часто

*8. Я чувствовала себя грустной или
   ☐ Да, все время
   ☐ Да, довольно часто
   ☐ Нет, не так часто
   ☐ Нет, никогда

*9. Мне было так плохо, что я плакала
   ☐ Да, почти все время
   ☐ Да, довольно часто
   ☐ Нет, очень редко
   ☐ Нет, никогда

*10 Мне приходило в голову сделать с собой что-то плохое
   ☐ Да, очень часто
   ☐ Нет, почти никогда
   ☐ Нет, почти никогда
   ☐ Нет, никогда

© The Royal College of Psychiatrists 1987.

161

Samoan

Ona o lea e te maito, pe lei leva atu foi ona e fanau, matou te fia iloa poo a ni ou lagona. Fa'amolemole siaki le tali e tali tutusa ma ou lagona o loo fa'alogoina I LE FITU ASO UA TEA, e le na o lagona o loo iai I le taimi nei.

O le fa'ataitaiga lea ua uma ona fai atu mo oe.

Na ou lagona le fiafia:
- ☐ Ioe I taimi uma lava
- ☐ Ioe I le tele o taimi
- ☐ Leai, e le o taimi uma
- ☐ Leai, matuai leai lava

O lona uiga: 'Ou te fa'alogoina le fiafia I le tele o taimi' I le vaiaso ua tuanai atu.

Fa'amolemole fa'atumu mai isi fesili I le auala lea e tasi.

I le 7 aso ua tea

1. Sa mafai ona ou ata ma ou iloa foi le malie o mea I nisi itu:
   - ☐ Tele lava pei ona masani ai
   - ☐ Tau le tupu I le taimi nei
   - ☐ Matuai le tupu lava
   - ☐ Matuai leai lava

2. Matuai ou fa'amoemoe lava ia maua le fiafia I mea e fai:
   - ☐ Sili atu nai le mea masani ai
   - ☐ Sili le maulalo nai le mea e masani ai
   - ☐ Manino e maulalo nai lo le mea masani ai
   - ☐ Seasea lava

3. E tele lava ina ou tuuaia fa'aletatau ia te au mea sese E tutupu:
   - ☐ Ioe, I le tele o taimi
   - ☐ Ioe, I nisi taimi
   - ☐ E le masani ai
   - ☐ Leai lava

4. Ou lagona le atuatuvale ma le popole ae leai se mafua'aga tatau:
   - ☐ Leai, matuai leai lava
   - ☐ Seasea lava
   - ☐ Ioe I nisi taimi
   - ☐ Ioe, e tupu soo

5. Ou te lagona le fefe ma le popole vale ae leai se mafua'aga tatau:
   - ☐ Ioe I le tele o taimi
   - ☐ Ioe, I nisi taimi
   - ☐ Leai, tau le tupu
   - ☐ Leai, e lei tupu lava

*6. Tele mea e saputu mai I luga o au:
   - ☐ Ioe,I le tele o taimi ua tele ina ou le lava tia I taimi uma
   - ☐ Ioe,I nisi taimi ua ou le gafatia nai lo le mea masani
   - ☐ Leai,ou te lavatia lava I taimi uma
   - ☐ Leai,o lea ou te mafaia lava mea uma pei ona masani ai

*7. Matuai ou fa'anoanoa lava ua tau le mafai ai ona ou moe:
   - ☐ Ioe,I le tele o taimi
   - ☐ Ioe, I nisi taimi
   - ☐ Tau le tupu soo
   - ☐ Matuai leai lava

*8. Ou te lagona le fa'anoanoa poo le le fiafia:
   - ☐ Ioe, I le tele o taimi
   - ☐ Ioe ae le tupu soo
   - ☐ Seasea
   - ☐ Leai e le o taimi uma

*9. Na o lou tagi soo I lou le fiafia:
   - ☐ Ioe, I le tele o taimi uma
   - ☐ Ioe, fai soo
   - ☐ E seasea
   - ☐ Leai, e lei tupu lava

*10. Na oo mai ia te au lagona e f'a'amanualia lou tino:
   - ☐ Ioe, tupu soo
   - ☐ Nisi taimi
   - ☐ E lei mafai lava
   - ☐ E lei tupu

Serbian

Како се осећате?

Пошто сте недавно родили бебу ми бисмо желели да знамо како се сада осећате. Молимо вас, <u>подвуците</u> одговор који најприближније описује како сте се осећали у последњих 7 дана, а не само како се данас осећате. Ево једног примера који је већ урађен:

Осећала сам се срећно:

Да, углавном
<u>Да, понекад</u>
Не, не тако често
Не, уопште не

Ово би значило "У току прошле недеље осећала сам се понекад срећно."

Молимо вас одговорите на остала питања на исти начин.

У последњих 7 дана

1. Могла сам да се смејем и да видим смешну страну свега:

    Исто као што сам и увек могла
    Не тако често сада
    Дефинитивно не тако често сада
    Уопште не

2. Све сам очекивала радосно и са уживањем:

    Исто као и пре
    Знатно ређе него пре
    Дефинитивно ређе него пре
    Скоро никад

3. Кривила сам себе када нешто није било у реду:

    Да, углавном
    Да, понекад
    Не тако често
    Не, никада

4. Била сам забринута или узрујана без икаквог разлога:

    Не, уопште не
    Скоро никад
    Да, понекад
    Да, врло често

5. Осећала сам се преплашено или панично без икаквог разлога:

    Да, врло често
    Да, понекад
    Не, не тако често
    Не, уопште не

6. Све ми је било тешко:

    Да, углавном нисам могла да изађем на крај
    Да, понекад нисам могла да изађем на крај као обично
    Не, углавном сам излазила на крај прилично добро
    Не, излазила сам на крај добро као и увек

7. Била сам толико несрећна да ми је било тешко да спавам:
        Да, углавном
        Да, врло често
        Не тако често
        Не, никада

8. Осећала сам се тужно или јадно:
        Да, углавном
        Да, врло често
        Не тако често
        Не, уопште не

9. Била сам толико несрећна да сам плакала:
        Да, углавном
        Да, врло често
        Само повремено
        Не, никада

10. Мисли о самоповреди су ми падале на памет:
        Да, веома често
        Понекад
        Скоро никад
        Никад

Slovenian

Kako se počutite?

Ker ste pred nedavnim dobili otročička, bi mi radi ugotovili kako se sedaj počutite. Prosimo da podčrtate odgovor, ki najbližje opiše kako ste se počutili ne samo danes, ampak zadnjih 7 dni. Tu je izpolnjen primer:

> Počutila sem se srečno:
> Ja, večinoma
> Ja, včasih
> Ne, ne preveč
> Ne, sploh ne

To bi pomenilo: 'Včasih med zadnjim tednom sem se počutila srečno'. Prosimo da izpolnite druga vprašanja na isti način.

V zadnjih 7 dneh

1. Uspelo mi je se nasmejati in videti smešno plat stvari:
   tako, kot mi je vedno uspelo
   manj kot prej
   veliko manj kot prej
   sploh ne

2. Veselila sem se stvari:
   tako, kot sem se vedno
   manj kot prej
   precej manj kot prej
   skoraj ne

3. Obremenjevala sem se, kadar so šle stvari narobe:
   ja, večino časa
   ja, nakaj časa
   redko
   ne, nikoli

4. Brez pravega razloga sem bila tesnobna in zaskrbljena:
   ne, sploh ne
   komaj kdaj
   ja, včasih
   ja, zelo pogosto

5. Brez pravega razloga sem se počutila prestrašeno in panično:
   ja, zelo pogosto
   ja, včasih
   redko
   ne, sploh ne

6. Stvari so se mi nakupičile:
   ja, večino časa jih nisem mogla obvladati
   ja, včasih jih nisem obvladala tako dobro kot prej
   ne, večino časa sem jih dobro obvladala
   ne, obvladala sem jih tako dobro kot vedno

7. Bila sem tako nesrečna, da sem slabo spala:
   ja, večino časa
   ja, precej pogosto
   redko
   ne, sploh ne

8. Počutila sem se žalostno ali nesrečno:
   ja, večino časa
   ja, precej pogosto
   redko
   ne, sploh ne

9. Bila sem tako nesrečna, da sem jokala:
   ja, večino časa
   ja, precej pogosto
   občasno
   ne, nikoli.

10. Pomislila sem, da bi si kaj naredila:
    ja, precej pogosto
    včasih
    skoraj nikoli
    nikoli

Somali

Maadaama aad mar dhawayd cunug dhashay, waxaan jeclaan lahayn inaan ogaano sida aad tahay. Fadlan HOOS KA XARIIQ jawaabta ugu dhow sida aad dareemeysay 7DII MAALMOOD OO LA SOO DHAAFAY, ma ahan sida aad maanta oo kaliya aad dareemaysid.

Kani waa tusaale la buuxiyey.

> Waxaan dareemayey farxad:
> Haa, mar kasta
> <u>Haa, inta badan</u>
> Maya, inta badan ma dareemeyn farax
> Maya, farax marnaba ma dareemeyn

Tan macnaheedu wuxuu noqonayaa: 'waxaan dareemayey farax wakhtiga intiisa badan' muddadii halka toddobaad ahayd ee la soo dhaafay. Fadalan u buuxi su'aalaha kale sidaas oo kale.

7 dii maalmood ee la soo dhaafay gudahooda

1. Waan qosli karay oo waxyaalaha dhinaca maaweelada ayaan ka arkayay:
   Sidii aan waligayba uga arki jiray
   Hadda sidii hore aad uma aha
   Shaki la'aan hadda sidii hore aad uma aha
   Haba yaraatee sidii hore ma aha

2. Waxaan si rajo fiican leh u sugayey inaan waxyaalaha ku raaxeysto:
   Sidii aan waligayba ugu sugi jirey
   In sidii hore xoogaa ka yar
   Shaki la'aan si sidii hore ka yar
   Haba yaraatee sidii hore ma ahan

*3. Si aan loo baahneyn ayaan naftayda isugu eedeynayey marka ay waxyaalo khaldamaan:
   Haa, inta badan
   Haa, mararka qaar
   Maya inta badan
   Maya, marnaba maya

4. Waan iska walaacsanaa iyadoo wax sabab ah oo weyn aysan jirin:
   Maya, haba yaraatee ma jirto
   In aad dirqi u ah
   Haa, marmar
   Haa, inta badan

*5.　Waxaan dareemayey cabsi iyo argagax iyadoo aan sabab weyn jirin:
　　　Haa, in aad u badan
　　　Haa, marmar
　　　Maya, in badan ma aha
　　　Maya, marnaba maya

*6.　Hawlahu ama waxyaalahu waa iga adkaanayeen:
　　　Haa, inta badan hawlaha ama arrimaha waan la qabsan waayey ama
　　　waan maamuli waayey gebi ahaanteedba
　　　Haa, mararka qaarkood hawlaha ama arrimaha waan la qabsan
　　　waayey ama waan u maamuli waayey sidii caadiga ii ahayd
　　　Maya, Inta badan si fiican ayaan ula qabsaday una maamuly
　　　Maya, waxaan ula qabsaday una maamulayey sidii aan waligay ahaa

*7.　Aad baan u farxad xumaa oo sidaa darteed seexashadu waa igu
　　　xumayd:
　　　Haa, wakhtiga intiisa badan
　　　Haa, mararka qaar
　　　Inta badan sidaa ma ahan
　　　Maya, haba yaraatee

*8.　Waxaan dareemayey murugaysnaan:
　　　Haa, wakhtiga intiisa badan
　　　Haa, marar badan
　　　Inta badan sidaa ma ahan
　　　Maya, haba yaraaatee

*9.　Aad baan u farxad xumaa sidaa darteed waan ooyayey:
　　　Haa, wakhtiga intiisa badan
　　　Haa, marar badan
　　　Mararka qaar oo kaliya
　　　Maya, marnaba maya

*10.　Fakar ah inaan naftayda waxyeelo ayaa igu soo dhacayey:
　　　Haa, in badan
　　　Marmar
　　　Si dirqi ah oo aad u yar
　　　Marnaba maya

South African (English)

As you have recently had a baby, we would like to know how you are feeling now. Please <u>underline</u> the answer that comes closest to how you feel. Please choose an answer that comes closest to how you have felt in the past seven days, not just how you feel today.

> For example, I have felt happy:
> Yes, all the time
> <u>Yes, most of the time</u>
> No, not very much
> No, not at all

This would mean: 'I have felt happy most of the time during the past week'.

In the past 7 days

1. I have been able to see the funny side of things:
   As much as I always could
   Not quite so much now
   Definitely not so much now
   Not at all

2. I have looked forward with enjoyment to things:
   As much as I ever did
   A little less than I used to
   Much less than I used to
   Hardly at all

3. I have blamed myself unnecessarily when things went wrong:
   Yes, most of the time
   Yes, some of the time
   Not very much
   No, never

4. I have been worried for no good reason:
   No, not at all
   Hardly ever
   Yes, sometimes
   Yes, very much

5. I have felt scared or panicky for no very good reason:
   Yes, quite a lot
   Yes, sometimes
   No, not much
   No, not at all

6. Things have been getting on top of me:
   Yes, most of the time I haven't been managing at all
   Yes, sometimes I haven't been managing as well as usual
   No, most of the time I have managed quite well
   No, I have been managing as well as ever

7. I have been so unhappy that I have had difficulty sleeping (not because of the baby):
   Yes, most of the time
   Yes, sometimes
   Not very much
   No, not at all

8. I have felt sad and miserable:
   Yes, most of the time
   Yes, quite a lot
   Not very much
   No, not at all

9. I have been so unhappy that I have been crying:
   Yes, most of the time
   Yes, quite a lot
   Only sometimes
   No, never

10. The thought of harming myself has occurred to me:
    Yes, quite a lot
    Sometimes
    Hardly ever
    Never

Spanish

¿Cómo se siente?

Como recientemente ha tenido un bebé, nos gustaría saber cómo se siente ahora. Por favor subraye la respuesta que considere más adecuada con respecto a cómo se ha sentido no sólo hoy, sino durante los últimos 7 días. A continuación encontrará un ejemplo ya completado.

Me he sentido bien:
Si, la mayoría del tiempo
Si, a veces
No, no muy bien
No, no me he sentido bien en absoluto

Esto significaría: 'Me he sentido bien en algunos momentos durante la semana pasada'. Por favor complete las otras preguntas de la misma manera.

En los pasados 7 días

1. He sido capaz de reírme y ver el lado divertido de las cosas:
   Igual que siempre
   Ahora, no tanto como siempre
   Ahora, mucho menos
   No, nada en absoluto

2. He mirado las cosas con ilusión:
   Igual que siempre
   Algo menos de lo que es habitual en mí
   Bastante menos de lo que es habitual en mí
   Mucho menos que antes

3. Me he culpado innecesariamente cuando las cosas han salido mal:
   Sí, la mayor parte del tiempo
   Sí, a veces
   No muy a menudo
   No, en ningún momento

4. Me he sentido nerviosa o preocupada sin tener motivo:
   No, en ningún momento
   Casi nunca
   Sí, algunas veces
   Sí, con mucha frecuencia

5. He sentido miedo o he estado asustada sin motivo:
   Sí, bastante
   Sí, a veces
   No, no mucho
   No, en absoluto

6. Las cosas me han agobiado:
    Sí, la mayoría de las veces no he sido capaz de afrontarlas
    Sí, a veces no he sido capaz de afrontarlas tan bien como siempre
    No, la mayor parte de las veces las he afrontado bastante bien
    No, he afrontado las cosas tan bien como siempre

7. Me he sentido tan infeliz que he tenido dificultades para dormir:
    Sí, la mayor parte del tiempo
    Sí, a veces
    No muy a menudo
    No, en ningún momento

8. Me he sentido triste o desgraciada:
    Sí, la mayor parte del tiempo
    Sí, bastante a menudo
    No con mucha frecuencia
    No, en ningún momento

9. Me he sentido tan infeliz que he estado llorando:
    Sí, la mayor parte del tiempo
    Sí, bastante a menudo
    Sólo en alguna ocasión
    No, en ningún momento

10. He tenido pensamientos de hacerme daño:
    Sí, bastante a menudo
    A veces
    Casi nunca
    En ningún momento

Spanish (USA)

Como usted hace poco tuvo un bebé, nos gustaría saber como se ha estado sintiendo. Por favor SUBRAYE la respuesta que más se acerca a como se ha sentido en los últimos 7 días.

OR

Por favor haga un círculo alrededor de la respuesta que más se acerca a como se ha sentido en los últimos 7 días.

Éste es un ejemplo ya completo:

Me he sentido contenta:
- 0 Sí, siempre
- 1 Sí, casi siempre
- 2 No muy a menudo
- 3 No, nunca

En los últimos 7 días

1. He podido reír y ver el lado bueno de las cosas:
   - 0 Tanto como siempre
   - 1 No tanto ahora
   - 2 Mucho menos
   - 3 No, no he podido

2. He mirado al futuro con placer:
   - 0 Tanto como siempre
   - 1 Algo menos de lo que solía hacer
   - 2 Definitivamente menos
   - 3 No, nada

3. Me he culpado sin necesidad cuando las cosas marchaban mal:
   - 3 Sí, casi siempre
   - 2 Sí, algunas veces
   - 1 No muy a menudo
   - 0 No, nunca

4. He estado ansiosa y preocupada sin motivo:
   - 0 No, nada
   - 1 Casi nada
   - 2 Sí, a veces
   - 3 Sí, a menudo

5. He sentido miedo o pánico sin motivo alguno:
   3 Sí, bastante
   2 Sí, a veces
   1 No, no mucho
   0 No, nada

6. Las cosas me oprimen o agobian:
   3 Sí, casi siempre
   2 Sí, a veces
   1 No, casi nunca
   0 No, nada

7. Me he sentido tan infeliz, que he tenido dificultad para dormir:
   3 Sí, casi siempre
   2 Sí, a menudo
   1 No muy a menudo
   0 No, nada

8. Me he sentido triste y desgraciada:
   3 Sí, casi siempre
   2 Sí, bastante a menudo
   1 No muy a menudo
   0 No, nada

9. He estado tan infeliz que he estado llorando:
   3 Sí, casi siempre
   2 Sí, bastante a menudo
   1 Sólo ocasionalmente
   0 No, nunca

10. He pensado en hacerme daño a mí misma:
    3 Sí, bastante a menudo
    2 Sí, a menudo
    1 Casi nunca
    0 No, nunca

Swedish

Hur mår Du?

Eftersom Du nyligen fått barn, skulle vi vilja veta hur Du mår. Var snäll och stryk under det svar, som bäst stämmer överens med hur Du känt Dig under de sista 7 dagarna, inte bara hur Du mår idag.

Här är ett exempel, som redan är ifyllt:

> Jag har känt mig lycklig:
> Ja, hela tiden
> Ja, för det mesta
> Nej, inte särskilt ofta
> Nej, inte alls

Detta betyder: Jag har känt mig lycklig mest hela tiden under veckan som har gått. Var snäll och fyll i de andra frågorna på samma sätt:

Under de senaste 7 dagarna

1. Jag har kunnat se tillvaron från den ljusa sidan:
   Lika bra som vanligt
   Nästan lika bra som vanligt
   Mycket mindre än vanligt
   Inte alls

2. Jag har glatt mig åt saker som skall hända:
   Lika mycket som vanligt
   Något mindre än vanligt
   Mycket mindre än vanligt
   Inte alls

3. Jag har lagt skulden på mig själv onödigt mycket när något har gått snett:
   Ja, för det mesta
   Ja, ibland
   Nej, inte så ofta
   Nej, aldrig

4. Jag har känt mig rädd och orolig utan egentlig anledning:
   Nej, inte alls
   Nej, knappast alls
   Ja, ibland
   Ja, mycket ofta

5. Jag har känt mig skrämd eller panikslagen utan speciell anledning:
   Ja, mycket ofta
   Ja, ibland
   Nej, ganska sällan
   Nej, inte alls

6. Det har kört ihop sig för mig och blivit för mycket:
   Ja, mesta tiden har jag inte kunnat ta itu med något alls
   Ja, ibland har jag inte kunnat ta itu med saker lika bra som vanligt
   Nej, för det mesta har jag kunnat ta itu med saker ganska bra
   Nej, jag har kunnat ta itu med saker precis som vanligt

7. Jag har känt mig så ledsen och olycklig att jar haft svårt att sova:
   Ja, mesta tiden
   Ja, ibland
   Nej, sällan
   Nej, aldrig

8. Jag har känt mig ledsen och nere:
   Ja, för det mesta
   Ja, rätt ofta
   Nej, sällan
   Nej, aldrig

9. Jag har känt mig så olycklig att jag har gråtit:
   Ja, nästan jämt
   Ja, ganska ofta
   Bara någon gång
   Nej,aldrig

10. Tankar på att göra mig själv illa har förekommit:
    Ja, rätt så ofta
    Ibland
    Nästan aldrig
    Aldrig

Tamil

1   வேடிக்கையான நிகழ்ச்சிகளை பார்த்து சிரிக்க முடியும்

அ. எப்பொழுதும் என்னால் முடிந்த அளவு
ஆ. எப்பொழுதாவது
இ. கண்டிப்பாக எப்பொழுதாவது

ஈ. முடியவே முடியாது

2   மகிழ்ச்சியான நிகழ்ச்சிகளுக்காக எதிர்நோக்கி கொண்டிருக்கிறேன்

அ. முடிந்த அளவு செய்திருக்கிறேன்

ஆ. முன்பைவிட சிறிது குறைந்துள்ளேன்

இ. கண்டிப்பாக முன்பைவிட குறைந்துள்ளேன்

ஈ. இல்லை

3   தவறான காரியங்கள் நிகழ்ந்த போது நான் என்னையே குறை கூறி உள்ளேன்

அ. ஆம். எல்லா நேரத்திலும்

ஆ. ஆம் சில நேரங்களில்

இ. எப்பொழுதாவது

ஈ. ஒருபோதும் இல்லை

4   தேவையற்ற காரணத்திற்காக நான் கவலைப்பட்டும், பயந்தும் உள்ளேன்

அ. இல்லவே இல்லை

ஆ. எப்பொழுதாவது

இ. ஆம் சில நேரங்களில்

ஈ. ஆம். அடிக்கடி

5   ஒன்றுமில்லாத காரணத்திற்காக பயந்த உணர்வும் மற்றும் பதட்ட உணர்வும்
அடைந்துள்ளேன்

அ. ஆம். நிறைய நேரம்

ஆ. ஆம். சிலநேரம்

இ. இல்லை எப்பொழுதாவது

ஈ. இல்லவே இல்லை.

6 என் மீது சுமை ∴ பாரம் அதிகரித்து உள்ளது.

   அ ஆம். நிறைய நேரங்களில் என்னால் எதிர்த்து சமாளிக்க முடிவதில்லை

   ஆ ஆம். சில நேரங்களில் என்னால் முன்பு மாதிரி சமாளிக்க முடிவதில்லை

   இ இல்லை. நிறைய நேரங்களில் நன்றாக சமாளித்து உள்ளேன்

   ஈ இல்லை. எப்பொழுதும் சமாளித்து உள்ளேன்.

7 தூக்கமின்மையால் நான் மகிழ்ச்சியாக இல்லை.

   அ ஆம். எல்லா நேரமும்
   ஆ ஆம். அடிக்கடி
   இ எப்பொழுதாவது
   ஈ இல்லவே இல்லை

8 துக்கமான மற்றும் மகிழ்ச்சியற்ற நிலையை உணர்ந்துள்ளேன்

   அ ஆம். எல்லா நேரமும்
   ஆ ஆம். அடிக்கடி
   இ எப்பொழுதாவது
   ஈ இல்லவே இல்லை

9 நான் அழுகையினால் சந்தோஷமின்றி இருக்கிறேன் ∴

   அ ஆம். எல்லா நேரமும்
   ஆ ஆம். அடிக்கடி
   இ எப்பொழுதாவது
   ஈ இல்லவே இல்லை

10 நான் என்னையே கொள்ளும் மனநிலையை அடைந்துள்ளேன்

   அ ஆம். எல்லா நேரமும்
   ஆ ஆம். அடிக்கடி
   இ எப்பொழுதாவது
   ஈ இல்லவே இல்லை

Thai

คุณกำลังรู้สึกอย่างไรบ้าง?

เนื่องจากคุณเพิ่งคลอดบุตรเมื่อเร็วๆ นี้ เราจึงอยากทราบว่าคุณกำลังรู้สึกอย่างไร โปรด<u>ขีดเส้นใต้</u>คำตอบที่ใกล้เคียงกับความรู้สึก
ของคุณในระยะ 7 วันที่ผ่านมา คือไม่ใช่ความรู้สึกเฉพาะวันนี้เท่านั้น ต่อไปนี้คือตัวอย่างการขีดเส้นใต้คำตอบ:

ฉันรู้สึกมีความสุข:

ใช่ เกือบตลอดเวลา
<u>ใช่ เป็นบางเวลา</u>
ไม่ ไม่ค่อยมีความสุข
ไม่ ไม่มีความสุขเลย

คำตอบนี้หมายความว่า "ฉันรู้สึกมีความสุขเป็นบางครั้งระหว่างสัปดาห์ที่แล้ว"

โปรดตอบคำถามต่อไปนี้ตามวิธีดังกล่าวข้างต้น:

ในระหว่าง 7 วันที่ผ่านมา

1. ฉันสามารถหัวเราะและมองดูสิ่งต่างๆ ในแง่ที่ขบขัน:

เท่าที่ฉันสามารถทำได้เสมอๆ
ตอนนี้ไม่สามารถทำได้มากหมือนอย่างที่เคยทำ
ตอนนี้ที่แน่ๆ คือไม่สามารถทำได้เหมือนอย่างที่เคยทำ
ไม่สามารถทำได้เลย

2. ฉันมองไปข้างหน้าเพื่อหาความแพลิดเพลินใจกับสิ่งต่างๆ:

เท่าๆ กับที่ฉันเคยทำ
น้อยลงกว่าที่เคยทำ
ที่แน่ๆ คือน้อยลงกว่าที่เคยทำ
เรียกได้ว่าเกือบไม่มีเลย

3. ฉันโทษตัวเองเมื่อมีเหตุการณ์เลวร้ายเกิดขึ้น:

ใช่ เกือบตลอดเวลา
ใช่ เป็นบางครั้ง
ไม่บ่อยนัก
ไม่เคยเลย

4. ฉันรู้สึกกระวนกระวายหรือกังวลโดยไม่มีเหตุผลสมควร:

ไม่ ไม่รู้สึกเช่นนั้นเลย
ไม่ค่อยจะรู้สึกเช่นนั้น
ใช่ เป็นบางครั้ง
ใช่ บ่อยมาก

5. ฉันรู้สึกหวาดผวาหรือตกอกตกใจโดยไม่มีเหตุผลสมควร:
    ใช่ บ่อยมากทีเดียว
    ใช่ เป็นบางครั้ง
    ไม่ ไม่บ่อยมาก
    ไม่ ไม่เคยเป็นเช่นนั้นเลย

6. มีเรื่องต่างๆ เกิดขึ้นทับถมฉันไปหมด:
    ใช่ ส่วนมากฉันไม่สามารถรับมือกับเรื่องเหล่านี้ได้เลย
    ใช่ บางครั้งฉันก็ไม่สามารถรับมือกับเรื่องเหล่านี้ได้เหมือนอย่างปกติ
    ไม่ ส่วนมากฉันสามารถรับมือกับเรื่องต่างๆได้ดี
    ไม่ ฉันสามารถรับมือกับเรื่องต่างๆได้เหมือนเช่นเคย

7. ฉันไม่มีความสุขเอามากๆ จนนอนไม่หลับ:
    ใช่ ส่วนมากเป็นเช่นนี้
    ใช่ เป็นเช่นนี้บ่อยทีเดียว
    ไม่ ไม่ค่อยเป็นเช่นนี้บ่อยนัก
    ไม่ ไม่เคยเป็นเช่นนี้เลย

8. ฉันรู้สึกเศร้าใจและไม่มีความสุข:
    ใช่ ส่วนมากเป็นเช่นนี้
    ใช่ เป็นเช่นนี้บ่อยทีเดียว
    ไม่ ไม่ค่อยเป็นเช่นนี้บ่อยนัก
    ไม่ ไม่เคยเป็นเช่นนี้เลย

9. ฉันไม่มีความสุขจนถึงกับต้องร้องไห้:
    ใช่ ส่วนมากเป็นเช่นนี้
    ใช่ เป็นเช่นนี้บ่อยทีเดียว
    เป็นบางครั้งเท่านั้น
    ไม่ ไม่เคยเป็นเช่นนี้เลย

10. ความคิดที่จะทำร้ายตัวเองเคยเกิดขึ้นกับฉัน:
    ใช่ เกิดขึ้นบ่อยทีเดียว
    เป็นบางครั้ง
    ไม่ค่อยจะเกิดขึ้น
    ไม่เคยเกิดขึ้นเลย

Turkish

Kendinizi nasıl hissediyorsunuz?

Yakın bir zamanda bebeğiniz oldu ve şimdi biz, kendinizi nasıl hissettiğinizi öğrenmek istiyoruz. Lütfen, yalnızca bugün değil, fakat son 7 gün içinde kendinizi nasıl hissettiğinizi en iyi tanımlayan ifadenin altını çiziniz, aşağidaki örnekte gösterildiği gibi:

> Mutlu hissettim:
> Evet, çoğu zaman
> Evet, zaman zaman
> Hayır, çok mutlu hissetmedim
> Hayır, hiç mutlu hissetmedim

Bunun anlamı şu olacak: 'Son bir hafta içinde kendimi ara sıra mutlu hissettim'. Lütfen diğer soruları da aynı şekilde cevaplandırınız.

Son 7 gündür

1. Gülebiliyor ve olayların komik tarafını görebiliyorum:
   Her zaman olduğu kadar
   Artık pek o kadar değil
   Artık kesinlikle o kadar değil
   Artık hiç değil

2. Geleceğe hevesle bakıyorum:
   Her zaman olduğu kadar
   Her zamankinden biraz daha az
   Her zamankinden kesinlikle daha az
   Hemen hemen hiç

3. Birşeyler kötü gittiğinde gereksiz yere kendimi suçluyorum:
   Evet, çoğu zaman
   Evet, bazen
   Çok sık değil
   Hayır, hiçbir zaman

4. Nedensiz yere kendimi sıkıntılı ya da endişeli hissediyorum:
   Hayır, hiçbir zaman
   Çok seyrek
   Evet, bazen
   Evet, çoğu zaman

5. İyi bir nedeni olmadığı halde, korkuyor ya da paniğe kapılıyorum:
   Evet, çoğu zaman
   Evet, bazen
   Hayır, çok sık değil
   Hayır, hiçbir zaman

6. Her şey giderek sırtıma yükleniyor:
   Evet, çoğu zaman hiç başa çıkamıyorum
   Evet, bazen eskisi gibi başa çıkamıyorum
   Hayır, çoğu zaman oldukça iyi başa çıkıyorum
   Hayır, her zamanki gibi başa çıkıyorum

7. Öylesine mutsuzum ki uyumakta zorlanıyorum:
   Evet, çoğu zaman
   Evet, bazen
   Çok sık değil
   Hayır, hiçbir zaman

8. Kendimi üzüntülü ya da çok kötü hissediyorum:
   Evet, çoğu zaman
   Evet, oldukça sık
   Çok sık değil
   Hayır, hiçbir zaman

9. Öylesine mutsuzum ki ağlıyorum:
   Evet, çoğu zaman
   Evet, oldukça sık
   Çok seyrek
   Hayır, asla

10. Kendime zarar verme düşüncesinin aklıma geldiği oldu:
    Evet, oldukça sık
    Bazen
    Hemen hemen hiç
    Asla

Twi

How are you feeling?
Sɛn na wote nka wɔ wo mu?

As you have recently had a baby, we would like to know how you are feeling now. Please choose the answer which comes closest to how you have felt in the past 7 days, not just how you feel today. Here is an example, already completed:

> I have felt happy:
> Yes, most of the time
> <u>Yes, some of the time</u>
> No, not very often
> No, not at all

This would mean: 'I have felt happy some of the time during the past week'. Please complete the other questions in the same way.

Wowoeɛ nnkyɛree biara nti yɛpɛ sɛ yɛhunu sedeɛ w'atenka teɛ seesei. Yɛsrɛ wo sɛ, mmuaeɛ a ɛne sedeɛ na w'atenka teɛ wɔ nna nson a atwam no ye pɛ no, yi baako mmom, ɛnnyɛ sedeɛ w'atenka teɛ ɛnne. Hwɛ nhwɛsoɔ nie:

> *M'ani agye:*
> *Aane, mprɛ pii*
> <u>*Aane, ɛtɔ berɛ bi a*</u>
> *Dabi, ɛnnyɛ mprɛ pii*
> *Dabi, m'ani nnye koraa*

Yei kyerɛ sɛ: Nnawɔtwe a atwam no, ɛyɛ a m'ani gye berɛ bi. Mesrɛ wo, bua nsɛmmisa a aka no saa ara.

In the past 7 days *Nna nson a atwam no*

1. I have been able to laugh and see the funny side of things:
   Matumi asere na mahunu deɛ ɛyɛ sere:
   As much as I always could *Sɛdeɛ metumi biara*
   Not quite so much now *Ɛnnyɛ bebree sɛ deɛ ɛte seesei*
   Definitely no so much now *Mehunu sɛ ɛnnte sɛ seesei*
   Not at all *Ɛnnte saa koraa*

2. I have looked forward with enjoyment to things:
   Mede anigyeɛ hwɛ deɛ ɛbɛsie no kwan:
   As much as I ever did *Sɛdeɛ metumi biara*
   Rather less than I used to *Ɛnnte sɛ deɛ na kane no meyɛ no*
   Definitely less than I used to *Mehunu sɛ ɛnnte sɛ deɛ na kane no meyɛ no*
   Hardly at all *Ɛyɛ den koraa sɛ m'ani bɛgye*

3. I have blamed myself unnecessarily when things went wrong:
   Mebɔ me ara me ho sommoɔ a ɛnnhia koraa wɔ nnooma a ɛnnkɔ yie ho:
   Yes, most of the time *Aane, mprɛ pii*
   Yes, some of the time *Aane, ɛtɔ berɛ bi a*
   Not very often *Ɛnnyɛ mprɛ pii*
   No, never *Dabi, ɛnnsii da*

4. I have been anxious or worried for no good reason:
    Me yam ahyehye me na nnɔɔma bi aha me a nnyinasoɔ biara nni mu:
      No, not at all *Dabi, ɛnnte saa koraa*
      Hardly ever *Eyɛ den sɛ ɛbɛsie*
      Yes, sometimes *Aane, ɛtɔ berɛ bi a*
      Yes, very often *Aane, mprɛ pii*

5. I have felt scared or panicky for no very good reason:
    Mebɔ hu anaa kakra bi pɛ na me yam ahyɛ me a ɛnni nnyinasoɔ biara:
      Yes, quite a lot *Aane, bɛyɛ sɛ mprɛ pii*
      Yes, sometimes *Aane, ɛtɔ berɛ bi a*
      No, not much *Dabi, ɛnnyɛ mprɛ bebree*
      No, not at all *Dabi, ɛnnte saa koraa*

6. Things have been getting on top of me:
    Nnɔɔma reyɛ aboro me so:
      Yes, most of the time I haven't been able to cope at all
      Aane, mprɛ pii no menntumi nnyɛ hwee koraa
      Yes, sometimes I haven't been coping as well as usual
      Aane, ɛtɔ berɛ bi a, menntumi nnyɛ hwee sɛdeɛ meyɛ no
      No, most of the time I have coped quite will
      Dabi, mprɛ pii no metumi yɛ deɛ ɛsɛ sɛ meyɛ
      No, I have been coping as well as ever
      Dabi, metumi yɛ deɛ ɛsɛ sɛ meyɛ sɛdeɛ meyɛ no daa no

7. I have been so unhappy that I have had difficulty sleeping:
    Madi awerɛhoɔ saa ara ma menntumi nna:
      Yes, most of the time *Aane, mprɛ pii*
      Yes, sometimes *Aane, ɛtɔ berɛ bi a*
      Not very often *Ɛnnyɛ mprɛ pii*
      No, not at all *Dabi, ɛnnte saa koraa*

8. I have felt sad or miserable:
    Me werɛ aho pa ara ma mayɛ basaa:
      Yes, most of the time *Aane, mprɛ pii*
      Yes, quite often *Aane, ɛtaa si*
      Not very often *Ɛnnyɛ mprɛ pii*
      No, not at all *Dabi, ɛnnte saa koraa*

9. I have been so unhappy that I have been crying:
    Me werɛ aho pa ara ma su ara na mesu:
      Yes, most of the time *Aane, mprɛ pii*
      Yes, quite often *Aane, ɛtaa si*
      Only occasionally *Berɛ bi pɔtee*
      No, never *Dabi, ɛnnsii da*

10. The thought of harming myself has occurred to me:
    Menyaa adwene bi sɛ mempira me ho:
      Yes, quite often *Aane, bɛyɛ sɛ mprɛ pii*
      Sometimes *Ɛtɔ da bi a*
      Hardly ever *Eyɛ den sɛ ɛbɛsi*
      Never *Ɛnnsii da*

Urdu

آپ کیسا محسوس کر رہی ہیں ؟

جیسا کہ تھوڑا عرصہ پہلے آپکے ہاں ولادت ہوئی ہے،ہم یہ جاننا چاہیں گے کہ اب آپ کیسا محسوس کر رہی ہیں ؟ مہربانی فرما کر اپنے جواب جو تقریبا آپکی حالت کے مطابق ہوں، کے نیچے سطر لگائیں کہ پچھلے سات دنوں سے آپکی طبعیت کیسی ہے نہ صرف یہ کہ آج کیسا محسوس کر تی ہیں. ذیل میں پہلے سے حل شدہ مثال دی جا رہی ہے.

میں نے اپنے آپکو خوش محسوس کیا ہے .
ہاں،کثر اوقات
<u>ہاں،بعض اوقات</u>
نہیں،بہت زیادہ نہیں
نہیں، بالکل نہیں

اس کا یہ مطلب ہو گا کہ" پچھلے ہفتے کے دوران میں نے بعض اوقات اپنے آپکو خوش محسوس کیا ہے". ازراہ کرم باقی سوالات کو اسی طرح مکمل کریں.

پچھلے سات دنوں سے

1. چیزوں کے مزاحیہ رخ کو دیکھ کر میں ہنسنے کے قابل تھی:

اتنا زیادہ جتنا پہلے ہنس سکتی تھی
اب اتنا زیادہ نہیں
یقینا اب کے اتنا زیادہ نہیں
بالکل نہیں

2. میں خوشی سے کسی چیز کے واقع ہونے کا انتظار کرتی ہوں:

اتنا زیادہ جتنا پہلے کیا کرتی تھی
پہلے سے قدرے کم
یقینا اس سے کم جتنا پہلے کیا کرتی تھی
بالکل بھی نہیں

3. جب کچھ غلط ہو جائے تو میں اپنےآپکو الزام دیتی ہوں:

اتنا ہی جتنا پہلے دیا کرتی تھی
اس سے قدرے کم جتنا پہلے دیا کرتی تھی
یقینا اس سے کم جتنا پہلے دیا کرتی تھی
نہیں،بھی نہیں

4. بغیر کسی معقول وجہ کے میں پریشان اور فکرمند رہی ہوں:

نہیں،بالکل نہیں
شاید ہی کبھی
ہاں،کبھی کبھار
ہاں،اکثر اوقات

5. میں نے بغیر کسی معقول وجہ کے خوف اور گھبراہٹ محسوس کی ہے:

ہاں، بہت زیادہ
ہاں، کبھی کبھار
نہیں، زیادہ نہیں
نہیں، کبھی نہیں

6. چیزیں میرے سر پر سوار رہی ہیں:

ہاں، اکثر اوقات میں کئی چیزوں کو نپٹانے میں ناکام رہی ہوں
ہاں، کبھی کبھی میں پہلے کی طرح چیزوں کو نپٹانے میں ناکام رہی ہوں
نہیں، میں اکثر اوقات چیزوں کو اچھی طرح نہیں نپٹا سکی
نہیں، میں پہلے کی طرح ہی خوش اسلوبی سے نپٹتی رہی ہوں

7. میں اتنی ناخوش رہی ہوں کہ مجھے سونے میں دشواری پیش آتی رہی ہے:

ہاں، زیادہ تر وقت
ہاں، اکثر اوقات
بہت زیادہ بار نہیں
نہیں، بالکل نہیں

8. میں نے خود کو غمگین اور افسردہ محسوس کیا ہے:

ہاں، زیادہ تر وقت
ہاں، اکثر اوقات
بہت زیادہ بار نہیں
نہیں، بالکل نہیں

9. میں اتنی زیادہ نا خوش رہی ہوں کہ میں روتی رہی ہوں:

ہاں، زیادہ تر وقت
ہاں، اکثر اوقات
صرف کبھی کبھار
نہیں، بالکل نہیں

10. خود کو نقصان پہنچانے کا خیال میرے دل میں پیدا ہوا:

ہاں، اکثر اوقات
کبھی کبھار
شاید ہی کبھی
کبھی نہیں

Vietnamese

Bạn cảm thấy thế nào?

Vì bạn vừa sinh cháu bé, nên chúng tôi muốn biết bạn cảm thấy thế nào. Xin gạch dưới câu trả lời nào phù hợp nhất với cảm giác của bạn trong 7 ngày qua, không phải chỉ hôm nay mà thôi. Sau đây là một thí dụ của câu trả lời:

> Bạn có cảm thấy vui vẻ không?
> Vâng, rất thường xuyên
> <u>Vâng, thỉnh thoảng</u>
> Không, không được vui lắm
> Không, không vui gì cả

Câu trả lời trên có nghĩa là: 'Thỉnh thoảng tôi cảm thấy vui vẻ trong suốt tuần qua'. Xin bạn trả lời những câu hỏi dưới đây theo cách chỉ dẫn trên.

Trong 7 ngày qua

1. Bạn vẫn có thể cười và thấy được phần hài hước của những chuyện khôi hài không?
   Vẫn như trước
   Bây giờ ít hơn trước
   Chắc chắn là ít hơn trước
   Không bao giờ như trước

2. Bạn có nhìn vào tương lai với niềm hân hoan/vui vẻ không?
   Vẫn như trước
   Ít hơn trước
   Chắc chắn là ít hơn trước
   Gần như không có

3. Bạn có tự đổ lỗi cho chính mình một cách quá đáng khi chuyện xảy ra không được như ý không?
   Rất thường xuyên
   Thỉnh thoảng
   Rất hiếm
   Không bao giờ

4. Bạn có cảm thấy không yên tâm hay lo sợ một cách vô lý không?
   Không bao giờ
   Rất hiếm
   Thỉnh thoảng
   Rất thường xuyên

5. Bạn có cảm thấy sợ sệt hay hoảng hốt một cách vô lý không?
   Vâng, nhiều lắm
   Vâng, đôi khi
   Không, rất hiếm
   Không khi nào

6. Bạn có cảm thấy mọi việc xảy ra đều quá sức chịu đựng của mình hay không?
   Vâng, thường xuyên tôi không thể giải quyết được bất cứ việc gì
   Vâng, thỉnh thoảng tôi không thể giải quyết được công việc như bình
   thường
   Không, thường xuyên tôi cũng có thể giải quyết được công việc như bình
   thường Không, tôi luôn luôn giải quyết công việc như bình thường

7. Bạn có cảm giác buồn đến mức khó ngủ không?
   Vâng, rất thường xuyên.
   Vâng, thỉnh thoảng
   Không thường lắm
   Không khi nào

8. Bạn có cảm thấy buồn hay khổ sở không?
   Vâng, rất thường xuyên
   Vâng, thỉnh thoảng
   Không thường lắm
   Không khi nào

9. Bạn có quá u buồn đến độ thường hay khóc không?
   Vâng, hầu như lúc nào cũng vậy
   Vâng, rất thường
   Không, không thường lắm
   Không khi nào

10. Bạn có bao giờ có ý nghĩ tự tử không?
    Vâng, rất thường
    Đôi khi
    Rất ít khi
    Không khi nào

Xhosa

Ngoku ndinemibuzo ekufuneka ndikubuze yona ngovakalelo lwakho lweveki ephelileyo. Nceda undinike impendulo esondele kakhulu kwindlela ozive ngayo EZINTSUKWINI EZISI-7 EZIGQITHILEYO, andilufuni uvakalelo lwakho lwanamhlanje.

1. Ndikwazile ukuhleka, ndakubona nokumangalisayo ezintweni.
   - ☐ Kangangoko bendikwenza ngaphambili
   - ☐ Hayi kangako, okwangoku
   - ☐ Ngokuqinisekileyo ayikho kangako okwangoku
   - ☐ Akunjalo

2. Ndikhe ndajonga phambili ndisonwatyiswa zizinto.
   - ☐ Kangangoko bendinokwenza
   - ☐ Kungaphantsi kunoko bendisenza
   - ☐ Ngokuqinisekileyo kungaphantsi kunoko bendisenza
   - ☐ Akwenzeki kwaphela

3. Ndizigxekile ngokungekho mfuneko xa izinto bezingahambi kakuhle.
   - ☐ Ewe, kumaxesha amaninzi
   - ☐ Ewe, ngamanye amaxesha
   - ☐ Akusoloko kusenzeka qho
   - ☐ Hayi, zange kwenzeke

4. Bendinexhala okanye ndikhathazekile kungekho sizathu.
   - ☐ Hayi, akunjalo
   - ☐ Zange kwenzeke
   - ☐ Ewe, ngamanye amaxesha
   - ☐ Ewe, kwenzeka qho

5. Ndizive ndibuhlungu okanye ndisoyika kungekho sizathu.
   - ☐ Ewe, kwenzeka kakhulu
   - ☐ Ewe, ngamanye amaxesha
   - ☐ Hayi, akwenzeki ngamandla
   - ☐ Hayi, akunjalo

6. Imeko ibindongamele.
   - ☐ Ewe, kumaxesha amaninzi bendingakwazi kumelana naloo nto
   - ☐ Ewe, ngamanye amaxesha bendingakwazi ukumelana naloo nto njengesiqhelo
   - ☐ Hayi, kumaxesha amaninzi bendimelana kakuhle naloo nto
   - ☐ Hayi, bendisoloko ndikwazi ukumelana naloo nto njengakuqala

7. Bendingonwabanga kunzima nokuba ndilale.
   - ☐ Ewe, kumaxesha amaninzi
   - ☐ Ewe, ngamanye amaxesha
   - ☐ Bekungenzeki qho
   - ☐ Hayi, akunjalo

8. Bendilusizi okanye bendixakanisekile.
   - ☐ Ewe, kumaxesha amaninzi
   - ☐ Ewe, ngamanye amaxesha
   - ☐ Bekungenzeki qho
   - ☐ Hayi, akunjalo

9. Bendingonwabanga ndada ndamana ndilila.
   - ☐ Ewe, kumaxesha amaninzi
   - ☐ Ewe, bekusoloko kusenzeka
   - ☐ Bekusenzeka kuphela ngamaxesha athile
   - ☐ Hayi, zange kwenzeke

10. Ikhe yandifikela ingcinga yokuba mandizenzakalise.
   - ☐ Ewe, bekusenzeka qho
   - ☐ Ngamanye amaxesha
   - ☐ Zange kwenzeke
   - ☐ Zange

References

Abiodun OA (2006) Postnatal depression in primary care populations in Nigeria. *General Hospital Psychiatry*, **28**, 133–136.

Adewuya AO (2006) Early postpartum mood as a risk factor for postnatal depression in Nigerian women. *American Journal of Psychiatry*, **163**, 1435–1437.

Adewuya AO, Ola BA, Dada AO, *et al* (2006) Validation of the Edinburgh Postnatal Depression Scale as a screening tool for depression in late pregnancy among Nigerian women. *Journal of Psychosomatic Obstetrics and Gynaecology*, **27**, 267–272.

Agoub M, Moussaoui D, Battas O (2005) Prevalence of postpartum depression in a Moroccan sample. *Archives of Women's Mental Health*, **8**, 37–43.

Ahmed HM, Alalaf SK, Al-Tawi NG (2012) Screening for postpartum depression using Kurdish version of Edinburgh postnatal depression scale. *Archives of Gynecology and Obstetrics*, **285**, 1249–1255.

Aitken P, Jacobson R (1997) Knowledge of the Edinburgh Postnatal Depression Scale among psychiatrists and general practitioners. *Psychiatric Bulletin*, **21**, 550–552.

Alvarado-Esquivel C, Sifuentes AA, Salas MC, *et al* (2006) Validation of the Edinburgh Postpartum Depression Scale in a population of puerperal women in Mexico. *Clinical Practice and Epidemiology in Mental Health*, **2**, 33.

American Psychiatric Association (1980) *Diagnostic and Statistical Manual of Mental Disorders (3rd edn) (DSM-III)*. APA.

American Psychiatric Association (1994) *Diagnostic and Statistical Manual of Mental Disorders (4th edn) (DSM-IV)*. APA.

American Psychiatric Association (2013) *Diagnostic and Statistical Manual of Mental Disorders (5th edn) (DSM-5)*. APA.

Ancill R, Hilton S, Carr T, *et al* (1986) Screening for antenatal and postnatal depressive symptoms in general practice using a microcomputer-delivered questionnaire. *Journal of the Royal College of General Practitioners*, **36**, 276–279.

Angeli N, Grahame K (1990) Screening for postnatal depression. *Midwife, Health Visitor and Community Nurse*, **26**, 428–430.

Appleby L (1991) Suicide during pregnancy and in the first postnatal year. *BMJ*, **302**, 137–140.

Appleby L, Gregoire A, Platz C, *et al* (1994) Screening women for high risk of postnatal depression. *Journal of Psychosomatic Research*, **38**, 539–545.

Appleby L, Warner R, Whitton A, *et al* (1997) A controlled study of fluoxetine and cognitive–behavioural counselling in the treatment of postnatal depression. *BMJ*, **314**, 932–936.

Areias ME, Kumar R, Barros H, *et al* (1996a) Comparative incidence of depression in women and men, during pregnancy and after childbirth. Validation of the Edinburgh Postnatal Depression Scale in Portuguese mothers. *British Journal of Psychiatry*, **169**, 30–35.

Areias ME, Kumar R, Barros H, *et al* (1996*b*) Correlates of postnatal depression in mothers and fathers. *British Journal of Psychiatry*, **169**, 36–41.

Ascaso-Terrén C, Garcia-Esteve L, Navarro P, *et al* (2003) Prevalence of postpartum depression in Spanish mothers: comparison of estimation by mean of the structured clinical interview for DSM-IV with the Edinburgh Postnatal Depression Scale. *Medicina Clinica*, **120**, 326–329.

Atkinson KA, Rickel AU (1984) Postpartum depression in primiparous parents. *Journal of Abnormal Psychology*, **93**, 115–119.

Aydin N, Inandi T, Yigit A, *et al* (2004) Validation of the Turkish version of the Edinburgh Postnatal Depression Scale among women within their first postpartum year. *Social Psychiatry and Psychiatric Epidemiology*, **39**, 483–486.

Bågedahl-Strindlund M, Monsen Borjesson K (1998) Postnatal depression: a hidden illness. *Acta Psychiatrica Scandinavica*, **98**, 272–275.

Ballard CG, Davis R, Cullen PC, *et al* (1994) Prevalence of postnatal psychiatric morbidity in mothers and fathers. *British Journal of Psychiatry*, **164**, 782–788.

Banerjee N, Banerjee A, Kriplani A, *et al* (2000) Evaluation of postpartum depression using the Edinburgh postnatal depression scale in evaluation of postpartum depression in a rural community in India. *International Journal of Social Psychiatry*, **46**, 74–75.

Barclay L, Kent D (1998) Recent immigration and the misery of motherhood: a discussion of pertinent issues. *Midwifery*, **14**, 4–9.

Barker W (1998) Let's trust our instincts. *Community Practitioner*, **71**, 305.

Barnett B, Lockhart K, Bernard D, *et al* (1993) Mood disorders among mothers of infants admitted to a mothercraft hospital. *Journal of Paediatric and Child Health*, **29**, 270–275.

Barnett BE, Matthey S, Boyce P (1999) Migration and motherhood: a response to Barclay and Kent (1998). *Midwifery*, **15**, 203–207.

Becht MC, Van Erp CF, Teeuwisse TM, *et al* (2001) Measuring depression in women around menopausal age: towards a validation of the Edinburgh Depression Scale. *Journal of Affective Disorders*, **63**, 209–213.

Beck AT, Ward CH, Mendelsohn M, *et al* (1961) An inventory for measuring depression. *Archives of General Psychiatry*, **4**, 53–63.

Beck CT, Gable RK (2001) Comparative analysis of the performance of the Postpartum Depression Screening Scale with two other depression instruments. *Nursing Research*, **50**, 242–250.

Bedford A, Foulds G (1978) *Delusions, Symptoms, States. State of Anxiety and Depression (Manual)*. National Foundation for Educational Research.

Benjamin D, Chandramohan A, Annie IK, *et al* (2005) Validation of the Tamil version of Edinburgh post-partum depression scale. *Journal of Obstetrics and Gynecology of India*, **55**, 242–243.

Bennett HA, Einarson A, Taddio A, *et al* (2004) Prevalence of depression during pregnancy: systematic review. *Obstetrics and Gynecology*, **103**, 698–709.

Benvenuti P, Ferrara M, Niccolai C, *et al* (1999) The Edinburgh Postnatal Depression Scale: validation for an Italian sample. *Journal of Affective Disorders*, **53**, 137–141.

Bergant AM, Nguyen T, Heim K, *et al* (1998) Deutschsprachige Fassung und Validierung der 'Edinburgh postnatal depression scale' [German language version and validation of the 'Edinburgh postnatal depression scale']. *Deutsche Medizinische Wochenschrift*, **123**, 35–40.

Berginka V, Kooistra L, Lambregtse-van den Berg MP, *et al* (2011) Validation of the Edinburgh Depression Scale during pregnancy. *Journal of Psychosomatic Research*, **70**, 385–389.

Berle JØ, Aarre TF, Mykletun A, *et al* (2003) Screening for postnatal depression. Validation of the Norwegian version of the Edinburgh Postnatal Depression Scale, and assessment of risk factors for postnatal depression. *Journal of Affective Disorders*, **76**, 151–156.

Bielawska-Batorowicz E (1995) *Determinanty Spostrzegania Dziecka przez Rodziców w Okresie Poporodowym* [*Determinants of the Perception of the Child by Parents in the Postpartum Period*]. Wydawnictwo Uniwersytetu Łódzkiego.

Bloch M, Schmidt PJ, Danaceau M, *et al* (2000) Effects of gonadal steroids in women with a history of postpartum depression. *American Journal of Psychiatry*, **157**, 924–930.

Boath E, Cox J, Lewis M, *et al* (1999) When the cradle falls: the treatment of postnatal depression in a psychiatric day hospital compared with routine primary care. *Journal of Affective Disorders*, **53**, 143–151.

Boath E, Henshaw C (2001) The treatment of postnatal depression: a comprehensive literature review. *Journal of Reproductive and Infant Psychology*, **19**, 215–248.

Boath EH, Major K, Cox JL (2003) When the cradle falls II: the cost-effectiveness of treating postnatal depression in a psychiatric day hospital compared with routine primary care. *Journal of Affective Disorders*, **74**, 159–166.

Boyce PM, Stubbs J, Todd AL (1993) The Edinburgh Postnatal Depression Scale: validation for an Australian sample. *Australian and New Zealand Journal of Psychiatry*, **27**, 472–476.

Brugha TS, Sharp HM, Cooper SA, *et al* (1998) The Leicester 500 Project. Social support and the development of postnatal depressive symptoms: a prospective cohort survey. *Psychological Medicine*, **28**, 63–79.

Brugha TS, Wheatley S, Taub NA, *et al* (2000) Pragmatised randomised trial of antenatal intervention to prevent postnatal depression by reducing psychosocial risk factors. *Psychological Medicine*, **30**, 1273–1281.

Brugha TS, Morrell CJ, Slade P, *et al* (2011) Universal prevention of depression in women postnatally: cluster randomized trial evidence in primary care. *Psychological Medicine*, **41**, 739–748.

Buist A, Condon J, Brooks J, *et al* (2006) Acceptability of routine screening for postnatal depression: an Australia-wide study. *Journal of Affective Disorders*, **93**, 233–237.

Bunevicius A, Kusminskas L, Bunevicius R (2009) Validation of the Lithuanian version of the Edinburgh Postnatal Depression Scale. *Medicina (Kaunas Lithuania)*, **45**, 544–548.

Campbell SB, Cohn JF (1997) The timing and chronicity of postpartum depression: implications for infant development. In *Postpartum Depression and Child Development* (eds L Murray, PJ Cooper), pp. 165–201. Guilford Press.

Carpiniello B, Pariante CM, Serri F, *et al* (1997) Validation of the Edinburgh Postnatal Depression Scale in Italy. *Journal of Psychosomatic Obstetrics and Gynaecology*, **18**, 280–285.

Chandran M, Tharyan P, Muliyil J, *et al* (2002) Post-partum depression in a cohort of women from a rural area of Tamil Nadu, India. Incidence and risk factors. *British Journal of Psychiatry*, **181**, 499–504.

Changetech (2010) *First web-based prevention of postpartum depression*. Changetech (http://archive-no.com/page/1530323/2013-03-02/http://www.changetech.no/en/content/f%C3%B8rste-forebygging-av-f%C3%B8dselsdepresjon-p%C3%A5-web).

Chaudron LH, Pies RW (2003) The relationship between postpartum psychosis and bipolar disorder: a review. *Journal of Clinical Psychiatry*, **64**, 1284–1292.

Chaudron LH, Szilagyi PG, Tang W, *et al* (2010) Accuracy of depression screening tools for identifying postpartum depression among urban mothers. *Pediatrics*, **125**, e609–e617.

Chibanda D, Mangezi W, Tshimaga M, *et al* (2010) Validation of the Edinburgh Postnatal Depression Scale among women in a high HIV prevalence area in urban Zimbabwe. *Archives of Women's Mental Health*, **13**, 201–206.

Clark G (2000) Discussing emotional health in pregnancy: the Edinburgh Postnatal Depression Scale. *British Journal of Community Nursing*, **5**, 91–98.

Clifford C, Day A, Cox J (1997) Women's health after birth. Developing the use of the EPDS in a Punjabi-speaking community. *British Journal of Midwifery*, **5**, 616–619.

Clifford C, Day A, Cox J, *et al* (1999) A cross-cultural analysis of the use of the EPDS in health visiting practice. *Journal of Advanced Nursing*, **30**, 655–664.

Coast E, Leone T, Hirose A, *et al* (2012) Poverty and postnatal depresson: a systematic mapping of the evidence from low and lower middle income countries. *Health and Place*, **18**, 1188–1197.

Community Practitioners' and Health Visitors' Association (2003) *Postnatal Depression and Maternal Mental Health: A Public Health Priority*. CPHVA.

Condon JT, Corkindale CJ (1997) The assessment of depression in the postnatal period: a comparison of four self-report questionnaires. *Australian and New Zealand Journal of Psychiatry*, **31**, 353–359.

Condon J (2006) What about Dad? Psychosocial and mental health issues for new fathers. *Australian Family Physician*, **35**, 690–692.

Cooper PJ, Murray L (1995) Course and recurrence of postnatal depression. Evidence for the specificity of the diagnostic concept. *British Journal of Psychiatry*, **166**, 191–195.

Cooper PJ, Murray L, Hooper R, *et al* (1996) The development and validation of a predictive index for postpartum depression. *Psychological Medicine*, **26**, 627–634.

Cooper PJ, Murray L (1997) The impact of psychological treatments of postpartum depression on maternal mood and infant development. In *Postpartum Depression and Child Development* (eds L Murray, PJ Cooper), pp. 202–221. Guilford Press.

Cooper PJ, Tomlinson M, Swartz L, *et al* (1999) Post-partum depression and the mother–infant relationship in a South African peri-urban settlement. *British Journal of Psychiatry*, **175**, 554–558.

Corney RH (1980) Health visitors and social workers. *Health Visitor*, **53**, 409–413.

Cornish AM, McMahon CA, Ungerer J, *et al* (2005) Postnatal depression and infant cognitive and motor development in the second postnatal year: the impact of depression chronicity and infant gender. *Infant Behavior and Development*, **28**, 407–417.

Cox JL, Connor Y, Kendell RE (1982) Prospective study of the psychiatric disorders of childbirth. *British Journal of Psychiatry*, **140**, 111–117.

Cox JL (1983) Postnatal depression: a comparison of African and Scottish women. *Social Psychiatry*, **18**, 25–28.

Cox JL, Rooney A, Thomas PF, *et al* (1984) How accurately do mothers recall postnatal depression? Further data from a 3-year follow-up study. *Journal of Psychosomatic Obstetrics and Gynaecology*, **3**, 185–189.

Cox JL (1986) *Postnatal Depression: A Guide for Health Professionals*. Churchill Livingstone.

Cox JL, Holden JM, Sagovsky R (1987) Detection of postnatal depression. Development of the 10-item Edinburgh Postnatal Depression Scale. *British Journal of Psychiatry*, **150**, 782–786.

Cox JL (1989) Postnatal depression: a serious and neglected postpartum complication. *Baillière's Clinical Obstetrics and Gynaecology*, **3**, 839–855.

Cox JL, Gerrard J, Cookson D, *et al* (1993) Development and audit of Charles Street Parent and Baby Day Unit, Stoke-on-Trent. *Psychiatric Bulletin*, **17**, 711–713.

Cox JL (1996) Perinatal mental disorder – a cultural approach. *International Review of Psychiatry*, **8**, 9–16.

Cox JL, Chapman G, Murray D, *et al* (1996) Validation of the Edinburgh Postnatal Depression Scale (EPDS) in non-postnatal women. *Journal of Affective Disorders*, **39**, 185–189.

Cox JL (1998) Patients as parents: possible impact of changing childbirth and faltering families. *Archives of Women's Mental Health*, **1**, 55–61.

Cox JL (1999) Perinatal mood disorders in a changing culture. A transcultural European and African perspective. *International Review of Psychiatry*, **11**, 103–110.

Cox JL (2007) Antenatal and postnatal mental disorder: dynamic and cultural perspectives. *International Journal of Psychotherapy, Psychoanalysis and Psychiatry*, **40**, 37–51, 219–220.

Cox JL (2012) Conceptual and treatment approaches for a revitalised health service and renewed person-centered perinatal psychiatry. *International Journal of Person Centered Medicine*, **2**, 109–113.

Coyle N, Jones I, Robertson E, *et al* (2000) Variation at the serotonin transporter gene influences susceptibility to bipolar affective puerperal psychosis. *Lancet*, **366**, 1490–1491.

Craig E, Judd F, Hodgins G (2005) Therapeutic group programme for women with postnatal depression in rural Victoria: a pilot study. *Australasian Psychiatry*, **13**, 291–295.

Cryan E, Keogh F, Connolly E, *et al* (2001) Depression among postnatal women in an urban Irish community. *Irish Journal of Psychological Medicine*, **18**, 5–10.

Cubison J, Munro J (2005) Acceptability of using the EPDS as a screening tool for depression. In *Screening for Perinatal Depression* (eds C Henshaw, S Elliott), pp. 152–161. Jessica Kingsley.

Cullinan R (1991) Health visitor intervention in postnatal depression. *Health Visitor*, **64**, 412–414.

Da-Silva VA, Moraes-Santos AR, Carvalho MS, *et al* (1998) Prenatal and postnatal depression among low income Brazilian women. *Brazilian Journal of Medical and Biological Research*, **31**, 799–804.

Danaher BG, Milgrom J, Seeley JR, *et al* (2012) Web-based intervention for postpartum depression: formative research and design of the MomMoodBooster program. *Journal of Medical Internet Research Protocols*, **1**, e18.

de Bruin G, Swartz L, Tomlinson M, *et al* (2004) The factor structure of the Edinburgh Postnatal Depression Scale in a South African per-urban settlement. *South African Journal of Psychology*, **34**, 113–121.

Dennis CL, Creedy DK (2004) Psychosocial and psychological interventions for preventing postpartum depression. *Cochrane Database of Systematic Reviews*, **4**, CD001134.

Dennis CL, Ross LE, Grigoriadis S (2007) Psychosocial and psychological interventions for treating antenatal depression. *Cochrane Database of Systematic Reviews*, **3**, CD006309.

Dennis CL, Allen K (2008) Interventions (other than pharmacological, psychosocial or psychological) for treating antenatal depression. *Cochrane Database of Systematic Reviews*, **4**, CD006795.

Dennis CL, Ross LE, Herxheimer A (2008) Oestrogens and progestins for preventing and treating postpartum depression. *Cochrane Database of Systematic Reviews*, **4**, CD001690.

Dennis CL, Hodnett E, Reisman HM, *et al* (2009) Effect of peer support on prevention of postnatal depression among high risk women: multisite randomised controlled trial. *BMJ*, **338**, a3064.

Department of Health (2012) *Press release: NHS pledges more support for women with postnatal depression*. Department of Health, 16 May.

Derogatis LR, Cleary PA (1977) Confirmation of the dimensional structure of SCL-90: a study in construct validation. *Journal of Clinical Psychiatry*, **33**, 981–989.

Des Rivières-Pigeon C, Seguin CL, Brodeur JM, *et al* (2000) The Edinburgh Postnatal Depression Scale: the validity of its Quebec version for a population low socioeconomic status mothers. *Canadian Journal of Community Mental Health*, **19**, 201–214.

Dragonas T, Golding J, Ignatyeva R, *et al* (eds) (1996) *Pregnancy in the Nineties: The European Longitudinal Study of Pregnancy and Childhood*. Sansom.

Drake E, Howard E, Kinsey E (2013) Online screening and referral for postpartum depression: an exploratory study. *Community Mental Health Journal*, Jan 3. [Epub ahead of print]

Eberhard-Gran M, Eskild A, Tambs K, *et al* (2001) The Edinburgh Postnatal Depression Scale: validation in a Norwegian community sample. *Nordic Journal of Psychiatry*, **55**, 113–117.

Edhborg M, Lundh W, Seimyr L, *et al* (2001) The long-term impact of postnatal depressed mood on mother–child interaction: a preliminary study. *Journal of Reproductive and Infant Psychology*, **19**, 61–71.

Edhborg M, Lundh W, Seimyr L, *et al* (2003) The parent–child relationship in the context of maternal depressive mood. *Archives of Women's Mental Health*, **6**, 211–216.

Edmondson OJ, Psychogiou L, Vlachos H, *et al* (2010) Depression in fathers in the postnatal period: assessment of the Edinburgh Postnatal Depression Scale as a screening measure. *Journal of Affective Disorders*, **125**, 365–368.

Ekeroma AJ, Ikenasio-Thorpe B, Weeks S, *et al* (2012) Validation of the Edinburgh postnatal depression scale (EPDS) as a screening tool for postnatal depression in Samoan and Tongan women living in New Zealand. *New Zealand Medical Journal*, **125**, 41–50.

Elliott SA, Sanjack M, Leverton T (1988) Parents groups in pregnancy: a preventive intervention for postnatal depression? In *Marshaling Social Support: Formats, Processes and Effects* (ed. BH Gottlieb), pp. 87–110. Sage Publications.

Elliott SA (1994) Uses and misuses of the Edinburgh Postnatal Depression Scale in primary care: a comparison of models developed in health visiting. In *Perinatal Psychiatry: Use and Misuse of the Edinburgh Postnatal Depression Scale* (eds J Cox, J Holden), pp. 221–232. Gaskell.

Elliott SA, Leverton TJ (2000) Is the EPDS a magic wand? 'Myths' and the evidence base. *Journal of Reproductive and Infant Psychology*, **18**, 296–307.

Elliott SA, Leverton TJ, Sanjack M, *et al* (2000) Promoting mental health after childbirth: a controlled trial of primary prevention of postnatal depression. *British Journal of Clinical Psychology*, **39**, 223–241.

Elliott SA, Gerrard J, Ashton C, *et al* (2001) Training health visitors to reduce levels of depression after childbirth: an evaluation. *Journal of Mental Health*, **10**, 613–625.

Escribà-Agüir V, Artazcoz L (2011) Gender differences in postpartum depression: a longitudinal cohort study. *Journal of Epidemiology and Community Health*, **65**, 320–326.

Evans J, Heron J, Francomb H, *et al* (2001) Cohort study of depressed mood during pregnancy and after childbirth. *BMJ*, **323**, 257–260.

Evins GG, Theofrastous JP, Galvin SL (2000) Postpartum depression: a comparison of screening and routine clinical evaluation. *American Journal of Obstetrics and Gynecology*, **182**, 1080–1082.

Fairbrother N, Woody SR (2008) New mothers' thoughts of harm related to the newborn. *Archives of Women's Mental Health*, **11**, 221–229.

Felice E, Saliba J, Grech V, *et al* (2004) Prevalence rates and psychosocial characteristics associated with depression in pregnancy and postpartum in Maltese women. *Journal of Affective Disorders*, **82**, 297–301.

Felice E, Saliba J, Grech V, *et al* (2006) Validation of the Maltese version of the Edinburgh Postnatal Depression Scale. *Archives of Women's Mental Health*, **9**, 75–80.

Fernandes M, Srinivasan K, Stein S, *et al* (2011) Assessing prenatal depression in the rural developing world: a comparison of two screening measures. *Archives of Women's Mental Health*, **14**, 209–216.

Field T (1998) Maternal depression effects on infants, and early interventions. *Preventive Medicine*, **27**, 200–203.

Field T, Diego MA, Hernandez-Reif M, *et al* (2004) Massage therapy effects on depressed pregnant women. *Journal of Psychosomatic Obstetetrics and Gynaecology*, **25**, 115–122.

Field T, Diego M, Hernandez-Reif M (2006) Prenatal depression effects on the fetus and newborn: a review. *Infant Behavior and Development*, **29**, 445–455.

Field T (2010) Postpartum depression effects on early interactions, parenting, and safety practices: a review. *Infant Behavior and Development*, **33**, 1–6.

Fisher JRW, Cabral de Mello M, Patel V, *et al* (2006) Maternal depression and newborn health. *Newsletter of the Partnership for Maternal, Newborn & Child Health*, **2**, 13.

Fisher JR, Wynter KH, Rowe HJ (2010) Innovative psycho-educational program to prevent common postpartum mental disorders in primiparous women: a before and after controlled study. *BMC Public Health*, **10**, 432.

Fisher SD, Kopelman R, O'Hara MW (2012) Partner report of paternal depression using the Edinburgh Postnatal Depression Scale-Partner. *Archives of Women's Mental Health*, **15**, 283–288.

Fitzgerald MH, Ing M, Ya TH, *et al* (1998) *Hear Our Voices: Trauma, Birthing and Mental Health among Cambodian Women*. Transcultural Mental Health Centre.

Flaherty JA, Gaviria FM, Pathak D, *et al* (1988) Developing instruments for cross-cultural psychiatric research. *Journal of Nervous and Mental Disease*, **176**, 257–263.

Flynn HA, Sexton M, Ratlif S, *et al* (2011) Comparative performance of the Edinburgh Postnatal Depression Scale and the Patient Health Questionnaire-9 in pregnant and postpartum women seeking psychiatric services. *Psychiatry Research*, **187**, 130–134.

Freeling P (1992) Implications for general practice training and education. In *The Prevention of Depression and Anxiety: The Role of the Primary Care Team* (eds R Jenkins, J Newton, R Young), pp. 57–68. HMSO.

197

Gair S (1999) Distress and depression in new motherhood: research with adoptive mothers highlights important contributing factors. *Child and Family Social Work*, **4**, 55–66.

Garcia-Esteve L, Ascaso C, Ojuel J, et al (2003) Validation of the Edinburgh Postnatal Depression Scale (EPDS) in Spanish mothers. *Journal of Affective Disorders*, **75**, 71–76.

Gaskin K, James H (2006) Using the Edinburgh Postnatal Depression Scale with learning disabled mothers. *Community Practitioner*, **79**, 1462–2815.

Gausia K, Hamadani JD, Islam MD, *et al* (2007) Bangla translation, adaptation and piloting of Edinburgh Postnatal Depression Scale. *Bangladesh Medical Research Council Bulletin*, **33**, 81–87.

Gavin N, Gaynes B, Lohr K, *et al* (2005) Perinatal depression: a systematic review of prevalence and incidence. *Obstetrics and Gynecology*, **106**, 1071–1083.

Gemmill AW, Leigh B, Ericksen J, *et al* (2006) A survey of the clinical acceptability of screening for postnatal depression in depressed and non-depressed women. *BMC Public Health*, **6**, 211.

Georgiopoulos AM, Bryan TL, Wollan P, *et al* (2001) Routine screening for postpartum depression. *Journal of Family Practice*, **50**, 117–122.

Gerrard J, Holden JM, Elliott SA, *et al* (1994) A trainer's perspective of an innovative training programme to teach health visitors about the detection, treatment and prevention of postnatal depression. *Journal of Advanced Nursing*, **18**, 1825–1832.

Ghubash R, Abou-Saleh MT, Daradkeh TK (1997) The validity of the Arabic Edinburgh Postnatal Depression Scale. *Social Psychiatry and Psychiatric Epidemiology*, **32**, 474–476.

Gibson J, McKenzie-McHarg K, Shakespeare J, *et al* (2009) A systematic review of studies validating the Edinburgh Postnatal Depression Scale in antepartum and postpartum women. *Acta Psychiatrica Scandinavica*, **119**, 350–364.

Glasser S, Barell V, Shoham A, *et al* (1998) Prospective study of postpartum depression in an Israeli cohort: prevalence, incidence and demographic risk factors. *Journal of Psychosomatic Obstetrics and Gynaecology*, **19**, 155–164.

Glavin K, Smith l, Sørum R, *et al* (2010) Supportive counselling by public health nurses for women with postpartum depression. *Journal of Advanced Nursing*, **66**, 1317–1327.

Glaze R, Cox JL (1991) Validation of a computerised version of the 10-item (self-rating) Edinburgh Postnatal Depression Scale. *Journal of Affective Disorders*, **22**, 73–77.

Goldberg DP, Cooper B, Eastwood MR, *et al* (1970) A standardised psychiatric interview for use in community surveys. *British Journal of Preventive Social Medicine*, **24**, 1–23.

Goldberg DP (1972) *The Detection of Psychiatric Illness by Questionnaires*. Oxford University Press.

Goldberg DP (1992) Early diagnosis and secondary prevention. In *Prevention of Depression and Anxiety in General Practice: The Role of the Practice Team* (eds R Jenkins, J Newton, R Young), pp. 33–39. HMSO.

Gordan RE, Gordan KK (1960) Social factors in prevention of postpartum emotional adjustment. *Obstetrics and Gynecology*, **15**, 433–438.

Gotlib IH, Whiffen VE, Mount JH, *et al* (1989) Prevalence rates and demographic characteristics associated with depression in pregnancy and the postpartum. *Journal of Consulting and Clinical Psychology*, **57**, 269–274.

Grace SL, Evindar A, Stewart DE (2003) The effect of postpartum depression on child cognitive development and behavior: a review and critical analysis of the literature. *Archives of Women's Mental Health*, **6**, 263–274.

Green JM, Murray D (1994) The use of the Edinburgh Postnatal Depression Scale in research to explore the relationship between antenatal and postnatal dysphoria. In *Perinatal Psychiatry: Use and Misuse of the Edinburgh Postnatal Depression Scale* (eds J Cox, J Holden), pp. 180–198. Gaskell.

Green JM (1998) Postnatal depression or perinatal dysphoria? Findings from a longitudinal community-based study using the Edinburgh Postnatal Depression Scale. *Journal of Reproductive and Infant Psychology*, **16**, 143–155.

Grote V, Torstein V, von Kries R, *et al* (2010) Maternal postnatal depression and child growth: a European cohort study. *BMC Pediatrics*, **10**, 14.

Guedeney N, Fermanian J (1998) Validation study of the French version of the Edinburgh Postnatal Depression Scale (EPDS). New results about use and psychometric properties. *European Psychiatry*, **13**, 83–89.

Guedeney N, Fermanian J, Guelfi JD, *et al* (2000) The Edinburgh Postnatal Depression Scale (EPDS) and the detection of major depressive disorders in early postpartum: some concerns about false negatives. *Journal of Affective Disorders*, **61**, 107–112.

Haga SM, Ulleberg P, Slinning K, *et al* (2012) A longitudinal study of postpartum depressive symptoms: multilevel growth curve analyses of emotion regulation strategies, breastfeeding self-efficacy, and social support. *Archives Women's Mental Health*, **15**, 175–184.

Halbreich U, Karkun S (2006) Cross-cultural and social diversity of prevalence of postpartum depression and depressive symptoms. *Journal of Affective Disorders*, **91**, 97–111.

Hamilton M (1960) A rating scale for depression. *Journal of Neurology, Neurosurgery and Psychiatry*, **23**, 56–62.

Hanlon C, Medhin G, Alem A, *et al* (2008) Detecting perinatal common mental disorders in Ethiopia: validation of the self-reporting questionnaire and Edinburgh Postnatal Depression Scale. *Journal of Affective Disorders*, **108**, 251–262.

Hanlon C (2012) Maternal depression in low and middle income countries. *International Health*, **5**, 4–5.

Hanusa BH, Scholle SH, Hudson S, *et al* (2008) Screening for depression in the postpartum period: a comparison of three instruments. *Journal of Women's Health*, **17**, 585–596.

Harris B, Huckle P, Thomas R, *et al* (1989) The use of rating scales to identify post-natal depression. *British Journal of Psychiatry*, **154**, 813–817.

Harrison M (1992) Linking with voluntary and community resources: Homestart consultancy. In *Prevention of Depression and Anxiety in General Practice: The Role of the Practice Team* (eds J Jenkins, R Newton, R Young), pp. 140–144. HMSO.

Hay DF, Pawlby S, Sharp D, *et al* (2001) Intellectual problems shown by 11-year-old children whose mothers had postnatal depression. *Journal of Child Psychology and Psychiatry*, **42**, 871–889.

Hearn G, Iliff A, Jones I, *et al* (1998) Postnatal depression in the community. *British Journal of General Practice*, **48**, 1064–1066.

Heh SS (2001) Validation of the Chinese version of the Edinburgh Postnatal Depression Scale: detecting postnatal depression in Taiwanese women. *Nursing Research (China)*, **9**, 105–113.

Hendrick V, Altshuler L, Strouse T, *et al* (2000) Postpartum and nonpostpartum depression: differences in presentation and response to pharmacologic treatment. *Depression and Anxiety*, **11**, 66–72.

Henshaw C (2003) Mood disturbance in the early puerperium: a review. *Archives of Women's Mental Health*, **6**, S33–S42.

Henshaw C, Foreman D, Cox JL (2004) Postnatal blues: a risk factor for postnatal depression. *Journal of Psychosomatic Obstetrics and Gynecology*, **25**, 267–272.

Henshaw C, Cox J, Barton J (2009) *Modern Management of Perinatal Psychiatric Disorders*. RCPsych Publications.

Herz E, Thoma M, Umek W, *et al* (1997) Non-psychotic postpartum depression. *Geburtshilfe und Frauenheilkunde*, **57**, 282–288.

Hewitt C, Gilbody S, Brealey S, *et al* (2009) Methods to identify postnatal depression in primary care: an integrated evidence synthesis and value of information analysis. *Health Technology Assessment*, **13**, 1–145.

Holden JM (1988) *Counselling by Health Visitors in the Treatment of Postnatal Depression*. MPhil thesis. Department of Psychiatry, University of Edinburgh.

Holden JM, Sagovsky RS, Cox JL (1989) Counselling in a general practice setting: a controlled study of health visitor intervention in the treatment of postnatal depression. *BMJ*, **298**, 223–226.

Holden J (1996) The role of health visitors in postnatal depression. *International Review of Psychiatry*, **8**, 79–86.

Holden JM (1991) Postnatal depression: its nature, effects, and identification using the Edinburgh Postnatal Depression Scale. *Birth*, **18**, 211–221.

Holopainen D (2002) The experience of seeking help for postnatal depression. *Australian Journal of Advanced Nursing*, **19**, 39–44.

Holt WJ (1995) The detection of postnatal depression in general practice using the Edinburgh Postnatal Depression Scale. *New Zealand Medical Journal*, **108**, 57–59.

Howard L, Hoffbrand S, Henshaw C, *et al* (2005) Antidepressant prevention of postnatal depression. *Cochrane Database of Systematic Reviews*, **2**, CD004363.

Howard LM, Flach C, Mehay A, *et al* (2011) The prevalence of suicidal ideation identified by the Edinburgh Postnatal Depression Scale in postpartum women in primary care: findings from the RESPOND trial. *BMC Pregnancy and Childbirth*, **11**, 57.

Jadresic E, Jara C, Miranda M, *et al* (1992) Tastornos emocionales en el embarazo y el peuerperio: estudio prospective de 108 mujeres [Emotional disorders in pregnancy and the puerperium: a prospective study of 108 women]. *Revista Chilena de Neuro-Psiquiatria*, **30**, 99–106.

Jadresic E, Araya R, Jara C (1995) Validation of the Edinburgh Postnatal Depression Scale (EPDS) in Chilean postpartum women. *Journal of Psychosomatic Obstetrics and Gynaecology*, **16**, 187–191.

Jennings KD, Ross S, Popper S, *et al* (1999) Thought of harming infants in depressed and nondepressed mothers. *Journal of Affective Disorders*, **98**, 274–279.

Johnstone SJ, Boyce PM, Hickey AR, *et al* (2001) Obstetric risk factors for postnatal depression in urban and rural community samples. *Australian and New Zealand Journal of Psychiatry*, **35**, 69–74.

Joint Commissioning Panel for Mental Health (2012) *Guidance for Commissioners of Perinatal Mental Health Services. Volume Two: Practical Mental Health Commissioning*. JCPMH.

Jomeen J, Martin CR (2007) Replicability and stability of the multidimensional model of the Edinburgh Postnatal Depression Scale in late pregnancy. *Journal of Psychiatric and Mental Health Nursing*, **14**, 319–324.

Jones I, Hamshere M, Nangle JM, *et al* (2007) Bipolar affective puerperal psychosis: genome-wide significant evidence for linkage to chromosome 16. *American Journal of Psychiatry*, **164**, 1099–1104.

Josefsson A, Berg G, Nordin C, *et al* (2001) Prevalence of depressive symptoms in late pregnancy and postpartum. *Acta Obstetricia et Gynecologica Scandinavica*, **80**, 251–255.

Kadir AA, Nordin R, Ismail SB, *et al* (2004) Validation of the Malay version of the Edinburgh Postnatal Depression Scale for postnatal women in Kelantan, Malaysia. *Asia Pacific Family Medicine*, **3**, 9–18.

Kaplan PS, Bachorowski J, Zarlengo-Strouse P (1999) Child-directed speech produced by mothers with symptoms of depression fails to promote associative learning in 4-month old infants. *Child Development*, **70**, 560–570.

Katzenelson SK, Maizel S, Zilber N, *et al* (2000) Validation of the Hebrew version of the Edinburgh Postnatal Depression Scale: methods, results and application. In *Abstracts of the Tenth Congress of the Israel Psychiatric Association, Jerusalem, April 2000* [in Hebrew], p. 163. Israel Psychiatric Association.

Kemp L, Harris E, McMahon C, *et al* (2013) Benefits of psychosocial intervention and continuity of care by child and family health nurses in the pre- and postnatal period: process evaluation. *Journal of Advanced Nursing*, **69**, 1850–1861.

Kendell RE, Rennie D, Clarke JA, *et al* (1981*a*) The social and obstetric correlates of psychiatric admission in the puerperium. *Psychological Medicine*, **11**, 341–350.

Kendell R, Maguire R, Connor Y, *et al* (1981*b*) Mood changes in the first three weeks after childbirth. *Journal of Affective Disorders*, **3**, 317–326.

Kheirabadi GR, Maracy MR, Akbaripour S, *et al* (2012) Psychometric properties and diagnostic accuracy of the Edinburgh Postnatal Depression Scale in a sample of Iranian women. *Iranian Journal of Medical Sciences*, **37**, 32–38.

Kim J, Buist A (2005) Postnatal depression: a Korean perspective. *Australasian Psychiatry*, **13**, 68–71.

Kit LK, Janet G, Jegasothy R (1997) Incidence of postnatal depression in Malaysian women. *Journal of Obstetrics and Gynaecology Research*, **23**, 85–89.

Kozinszky Z, Dudas RB, Devosa I, *et al* (2012) Can a brief antepartum preventive group intervention help reduce postpartum depressive symptomatology? *Psychotherapy and Psychosomatics*, **81**, 98–107.

Kumar R, Robson K (1978) Neurotic disturbance during pregnancy and the puerperium; preliminary report of a prospective survey of 119 primiparae. In *Mental Illness in Pregnancy and the Puerperium* (ed. M Sandler), pp. 40–51. Oxford University Press.

Kumar R (1982) Neurotic disorders in childbearing women. In *Motherhood and Mental Illness* (eds I Brockington, R Kumar), pp. 71–118. Academic Press.

Kumar R (1994) Postnatal mental illness: a transcultural perspective. *Social Psychiatry and Psychiatric Epidemiology*, **29**, 250–264.

Lai BPY, Tang AKL, Lee DTS, *et al* (2010) Detecting postnatal depression in Chinese men: a comparison of three instruments. *Psychiatry Research*, **180**, 80–85.

Lam N, Contreras H, Mori E, *et al* (2009) Comparison of two self report questionnaires for depressive symptoms detection in pregnant women. *Anales de la Facultidad Medecina*, **80**, 28–32.

Lau Y, Wang Y, Lei Y, *et al* (2010) Validation of the Mainland Chinese version of the Edinburgh Postnatal Depression Scale in Chengdu mothers. *International Journal of Nursing Studies*, **47**, 1139–1151.

Laungani P (2000) Postnatal depression across cultures: conceptual and methodological considerations. *International Journal of Health Promotion and Education*, **38**, 86–94.

Lawrie TA, Hofmeyr GJ, De Jager M, *et al* (1998) Validation of the Edinburgh Postnatal Depression Scale on a cohort of South African women. *South African Medical Journal*, **88**, 1340–1344.

Lee DT, Wong CK, Ungvari GS, *et al* (1997) Screening psychiatric morbidity after miscarriage: application of the 30-item General Health Questionnaire and the Edinburgh Postnatal Depression Scale. *Psychosomatic Medicine*, **59**, 207–210.

Lee DT, Yip SK, Chiu HF, *et al* (1998) Detecting postnatal depression in Chinese women. Validation of the Chinese version of the Edinburgh Postnatal Depression Scale. *British Journal of Psychiatry*, **172**, 433–437.

Leonardou AA, Zervas YM, Papageorgiou CC, *et al* (2009) Validation of the Edinburgh Postnatal Depression Scale and prevalence of postnatal depression at two months postpartum in a sample of Greek mothers. *Journal of Reproductive and Infant Psychology*, **27**, 28–39.

Leviston A, Downs M (1999) Open space. When instinct is not enough. *Community Practitioner*, **72**, 184–185.

Lewinsohn PM, Antonuccio DO, Steinmetz JL, *et al* (1984) *The Coping with Depression Course: A Psycho-Educational Intervention for Unipolar Depression*. Castalsa.

Lloyd-Williams M, Friedman T, Rudd N (2000) Criterion validation of the Edinburgh Postnatal Depression Scale as a screening tool for depression in patients with advanced metastatic cancer. *Journal of Pain and Symptom Management*, **20**, 259–265.

Logsdon MC, Hutti MH (2006) Readability: an important issue impacting healthcare for women with postpartum depression. *American Journal of Maternal Child Nursing*, **31**, 350–355.

Logsdon MC, Myers JA (2010) Comparative performance of two depression screening instruments in adolescent mothers. *Journal of Women's Health*, **19**, 1123–1128.

Lundh W, Gyllang C (1993) Use of the Edinburgh Postnatal Depression Scale in some Swedish child health care centres. *Scandinavian Journal of Caring Sciences*, **7**, 149–154.

Lussier V, David H, Saucier J-F, *et al* (1996) Self-rating assessment of postnatal depression: a comparison of the Beck Depression Inventory and the Edinburgh Postnatal Depression Scale. *Pre- and Peri-Natal Psychology Journal*, **11**, 81–91.

MacArthur C, Winter HR, Bick DE, *et al* (2002) Effects of redesigned community postnatal care on women's health 4 months after birth: a cluster randomised controlled trial. *Lancet*, **359**, 378–385.

Madsen S (2006) *Becoming a Father: Men's Reactions to Parenthood*. Rigshospitalet.

Mahmud WMRW, Awang A, Mohammad MZ (2003) Revalidation of the Malay version of the Edinburgh postnatal depression scale (EPDS) among Malay postnatal women attending the Bakar Bata Health Center in Alor Setar, Kedah, North West of Peninsular Malaysia. *Malaysian Journal of Medical Sciences*, **10**, 71–75.

Malan DH, Heath ES, Bacal HA, *et al* (1975) Psychodynamic changes in untreated neurotic patients – II. Apparently genuine improvements. *Archives of General Psychiatry*, **32**, 110–126.

Mathers CD, Looncar D (2006) Projections of global mortality and Burden of Disease from 2002 to 2030. *PLoS Med*, **3**, 2011–2031.

Matthey S, Barnett BE, Elliott A (1997) Vietnamese and Arabic women's responses to the Diagnostic Interview Schedule (depression) and self-report questionnaires: cause for concern. *Australian and New Zealand Journal of Psychiatry*, **31**, 360–369.

Matthey S, Barnett BE, Kavanagh DJ, *et al* (2001) Validation of the Edinburgh Postnatal Depression Scale for men, and comparison of item endorsement with their partners. *Journal of Affective Disorders*, **64**, 175–184.

Matthey S (2004) Calculating clinically significant change in postnatal depression studies using the Edinburgh Postnatal Depression Scale. *Journal of Affective Disorders*, **78**, 269–272.

Matthey S, Kavanagh DJ, Howie P, *et al* (2004) Prevention of postnatal distress or depression: an evaluation of an intervention at preparation for parenthood classes. *Journal of Affective Disorders*, **79**, 113–126.

Matthey S, Henshaw C, Elliott S, *et al* (2006) Variability in use of cut-off scores and formats on the Edinburgh Postnatal Depression Scale: implications for clinical and research practice. *Archives of Women's Mental Health*, **9**, 309–315.

Matthey S, Ross-Hamid C (2012) Repeat testing on the Edinburgh Depression Scale and the HADS-A in pregnancy: differentiating between transient and enduring distress. *Journal of Affective Disorders*, **141**, 213–221.

Matthey S, Fisher J, Rowe H (2013a) Using the Edinburgh postnatal depression scale to screen for anxiety disorders: conceptual and methodological considerations. *Journal of Affective Disorders*, **146**, 224–230.

Matthey S, Lee C, Crnec R, *et al* (2013b) Errors in scoring the Edinburgh Postnatal Depression scale. *Archives of Women's Mental Health*, **16**, 117–122.

McCoy SJ, Beal JM, Peyton ME, *et al* (2005) Correlations of visual analog scales with Edinburgh Postnatal Depression Scale. *Journal of Affective Disorders*, **86**, 295–297.

McNair DM, Lorr M (1964) An analysis of mood in neurotics. *Journal of Abnormal and Social Psychology*, **69**, 620–627.

Mead N, Bower P, Gask L (1997) Emotional problems in primary care: what is the potential for increasing the role of nurses? *Journal of Advanced Nursing*, **26**, 879–890.

Milgrom J, Martin PR, Negri LM (1999) *Treating Postnatal Depression*. John Wiley & Sons.

Milgrom J, Gemmill AW, Bilszta JL, *et al* (2008) Antenatal risk factors for postnatal depression: a large prospective study. *Journal of Affective Disorders*, **108**, 147–157.

Milgrom J, Holt CJ, Gemmill AW, *et al* (2011) Treating postnatal depressive symptoms in primary care: a randomised controlled trial of GP management, with and without adjunctive counselling. *BMC Psychiatry*, **11**, 95.

Misri S, Kostaras X, Fox D, *et al* (2000) The impact of partner support in the treatment of postpartum depression. *Canadian Journal of Psychiatry*, **45**, 554–558.

Montazeri A, Torkan B, Omvidari S (2007) The Edinburgh Postnatal Depression Scale EPDS: translation and validation study of the Iranian version. *BMC Psychiatry*, **7**, 11.

Moore D, Ayers S (2011) A review of postnatal mental health websites: help for healthcare professionals and patients. *Archives of Women's Mental Health*, **14**, 443–452.

Moran TE, O'Hara MW (2006) A partner-rating scale of postpartum depression: the Edinburgh Postnatal Depression Scale – Partner (EPDS-P). *Archives of Women's Mental Health*, **9**, 173–180.

Morgan M, Matthey S, Barnett B, *et al* (1997) A group programme for postnatally distressed women and their partners. *Journal of Advanced Nursing*, **26**, 913–920.

Morrell CJ, Slade P, Warner R, *et al* (2009) Clinical effectiveness of health visitor training in psychologically informed approaches for depression in postnatal women: pragmatic cluster randomised trial in primary care. *BMJ*, **338**, a3045.

Murray D, Cox JL (1990) Identifying depression during pregnancy with the Edinburgh Postnatal Depression Scale (EPDS). *Journal of Reproductive and Infant Psychology*, **8**, 99–107.

Murray D, Cox JL, Chapman G, *et al* (1995) Childbirth: life event or start of a long-term difficulty? Further data from the Stoke-on-Trent controlled study of postnatal depression. *British Journal of Psychiatry*, **166**, 595–600.

Murray L, Carothers AD (1990) The validation of the Edinburgh Post-natal Depression Scale on a community sample. *British Journal of Psychiatry*, **157**, 288–290.

Murray L, Fiori-Cowley A, Hooper R, *et al* (1996) The impact of postnatal depression and associated adversity on early mother–infant interactions and later infant outcome. *Child Development*, **67**, 2512–2526.

Murray L, Cooper PJ, Wilson A, *et al* (2003) Controlled trial of the short- and long-term effect of psychological treatment of post-partum depression: 2. Impact on the mother–child relationship and child outcome. *British Journal of Psychiatry*, **182**, 420–427.

Muzik M, Klier CM, Rosenblum KL, *et al* (2000) Are commonly used self-report inventories suitable for screening postpartum depression and anxiety disorders? *Acta Psychiatrica Scandinavica*, **102**, 71–73.

National Institute for Health and Clinical Excellence (2007) *Antenatal and Postnatal Mental Health: Clinical Management and Service Guidance*. NICE.

National Institute for Health and Clinical Excellence (2009) *Depression in Adults: The Treatment and Management of Depression in Adults*. NICE.

Navarro P, Ascaso C, Garcia EL, *et al* (2007) Postnatal psychiatric morbidity: a validation study of the GHQ-12 and the EPDS as screening tools. *General Hospital Psychiatry*, **29**, 1–7.

Nielsen Forman D, Videbech P, Hedegaard M, *et al* (2000) Postpartum depression: identification of women at risk. *British Journal of Obstetrics and Gynaecology*, **107**, 1210–1217.

Oakley A (1980) *Women Confined: Towards a Sociology of Childbirth*. Martin Robertson.

Oates M (2001) Deaths from psychiatric causes. In *Why Mothers Die 1997–1999: The Confidential Enquiries into Maternal Deaths in the United Kingdom* (eds G Lewis, J Drife), pp. 65–187. Royal College of Gynaecologists and Obstetricians.

Oates M (2003) Suicide: the leading cause of maternal death. *British Journal of Psychiatry*, **183**, 279–281.

Oates MR, Cox JL, Neema S, *et al* (2004) Postnatal depression across countries and cultures: a qualitative study. *British Journal of Psychiatry*, **184**, s10–s16.

O'Hara MW, Zakoski EM, Philipps LH, *et al* (1990) Controlled prospective study of postpartum mood disorders: comparison of childbearing and nonchildbearing women. *Journal of Abnormal Psychology*, **99**, 3–15.

O'Hara MW (1994) Postpartum depression: identification and measurement in a cross-cultural context. In *Perinatal Psychiatry: Use and Misuse of the Edinburgh Postnatal Depression Scale* (eds J Cox, J Holden), pp. 145–168. Gaskell.

O'Hara MW (1995) *Postpartum Depression: Causes and Consequences*. Springer.

O'Hara MW, Stuart S, Gorman L, *et al* (2000) Efficiency of interpersonal psychotherapy for postpartum depression. *Archives of General Psychiatry*, **57**, 1039–1045.

Okano T, Murata M, Masuji F, *et al* (1996) Validation and reliability of a Japanese version of the EPDS. *Archives of Psychiatric Diagnosis and Clinical Evaluation*, **7**, 525–533.

Okano T, Nagata S, Hasegawa M, *et al* (1998) Effectiveness of antenatal education about postnatal depression: a comparison of two groups of Japanese mothers. *Journal of Mental Health*, **7**, 191–198.

Okano T, Sugiyama T, Nishiguchi H (2005) Screening for postnatal depression: validation of the EPDS and intervention period in Japanese health care system. Presented at The Australasian Marcé Society 2005 Conference, 8–10 September, Melbourne, Australia (http://www.marcesociety.com.au/marce/docs/BookletMarce2005.pdf).

Olioff M (1991) The application of cognitive therapy to postnatal depression. In *The Challenge of Cognitive Therapy: Applications to Non-Traditional Populations* (eds TM Vallis, JL Howes, PC Miller), pp. 111–133. Plenum Press.

O'Mahen H (2012) *University and Netmums join forces to tackle postnatal depression.* University of Exeter. Available at http://www.exeter.ac.uk/news/research/title_174561_en.html.

Onozawa K, Glover V, Adams D, *et al* (2001) Infant massage improves mother–infant interaction for mothers with postnatal depression. *Journal of Affective Disorders*, **63**, 201–207.

Ormel H, Koeter M, Van Der Brink W, *et al* (1990) The extent of non-recognition of mental problems in primary care and its effect on management and outcome. In *The Public Health Impact of Mental Disorder* (eds D Goldberg, D Tantum), pp. 154–165. Hogrefe and Huber.

Pace C (1992) A health education library in general practice. In *The Prevention of Depression and Anxiety: The Role of the Primary Care Team* (eds R Jenkins, J Newton, R Young), pp. 131–135. HMSO.

Painter A (1995) Health visitor identification of postnatal depression. *Health Visitor*, **68**, 138–140.

Patel V, DeSouza N, Rodrigues M (2003) Postnatal depression and infant growth and development in low income countries: a cohort study from Goa, India. *Archives of Disease in Childhood*, **88**, 34–37.

Paulden M, Palmer S, Hewitt C, *et al* (2009) Screening for postnatal depression in primary care: cost effectiveness analysis. *BMJ*, **339**, b5203.

Paulson JF, Dauber S, Leiferman JA (2006) Individual and combined effects of postpartum depression in mothers and fathers on parenting behavior. *Pediatrics*, **118**, 659–668.

Paulson JF, Bazemore SD (2010) Prenatal and postpartum depression in fathers and its association with maternal depression: a meta-analysis. *Journal of the American Medical Association*, **303**, 1961–1969.

Pitanupong J, Liabsuetrakul T, Vittayanont A, *et al* (2007) Validation of the Thai Edinburgh Postnatal Depression Scale for screening postpartum depression. *Psychiatry Research*, **149**, 253–259.

Pitt B (1968) 'Atypical' depression following childbirth. *British Journal of Psychiatry*, **114**, 1325–1335.

Pollock JI, Manaseki HS, Patel V (2006) Detection of depression in women of child-bearing age in non-Western cultures: a comparison of the Edinburgh Postnatal Depression Scale and the Self-Reporting Questionnaire-20 in Mongolia. *Journal of Affective Disorders*, **92**, 267–271.

Poobalan AS, Aucott LS, Ross L, *et al* (2007) Effects of treating postnatal depression on mother–infant interaction and child development. Systematic review. *British Journal of Psychiatry*, **191**, 378–386.

Pop VJ, Komproe IH, Van Somm MJ (1992) Characteristics of the Edinburgh Postnatal Depression Scale in the Netherlands. *Journal of Affective Disorders*, **26**, 105–110.

Radloff LS (1977) The CES–D Scale: a self-report depression scale for research in the general population. *Applied Psychological Measures*, **1**, 385–401.

Rahman A, Iqbal Z, Lovel H, *et al* (2005) Screening for postnatal depression in the developing world: a comparison of the WHO self-reporting questionnaire (SRQ20) and the Edinburgh postnatal depression screen (EPDS). *Journal of the Pakistan Psychiatric Society*, **2**, 69.

Rahman A, Fisher J, Bower P, *et al* (2013) Interventions for common perinatal mental disorders in women in low- and middle-income countries: a systematic review and meta-analysis. *Bulletin of the World Health Organization*, **91**, 593–601.

Ramchandani PG, Stein A, O'Connor TG, *et al* (2008) Depression in men in the postnatal period and later child psychopathology: a population cohort study. *Journal of the American Academy of Child and Adolescent Psychiatry*, **47**, 390–398.

Ramchandani PG, Psychogiou L, Vlachos H, *et al* (2011) Paternal depression: an examination of its links with father, child and family functioning in the postnatal period. *Depression and Anxiety*, **28**, 471–477.

Reck C, Stehle E, Reinig K, *et al* (2009) Maternity blues as a predictor of DSM-IV depression and anxiety disorders in the first three months postpartum. *Journal of Affective Disorders*, **113**, 77–87.

Regmi S, Sligl W, Carter D, *et al* (2002) A controlled study of postpartum depression among Nepalese women: validation of the Edinburgh Postpartum Depression Scale in Kathmandu. *Tropical Medicine and International Health*, **7**, 378–382.

Rhandawa JK, Roach RR, Tareen SR, *et al* (2009) Validation study of Edinburgh Postnatal Depression Scale in Madagascar. *American Journal of Tropical Medicine and Hygiene*, **81**, 103.

Robertson E, Sherry G, Wallington T, *et al* (2004) Antenatal risk factors for postpartum depression: a synthesis of recent literature. *General Hospital Psychiatry*, **26**, 289–295.

Rowel D, Jayawardena P, Fernando N (2008) Validation of Sinhala translation of Edinburgh Postnatal Depression Scale. *Ceylon Medical Journal*, **53**, 10–13.

Roy A, Gang P, Cole K, *et al* (1993) Use of Edinburgh Postnatal Depression Scale in a North American population. *Progress in Neuro-Psychopharmacology and Biological Psychiatry*, **17**, 501–504.

Rubertsson C, Borjesson K, Berglaund A, *et al* (2011) The Swedish validation of Edinburgh Postnatal Depression Scale (EPDS) during pregnancy. *Nordic Journal of Psychiatry*, **65**, 414–418.

Rushidi WM, Azidah AK, Shaiful Bahari I, *et al* (2002) Validation of the Malay version of the Edinburgh Postnatal Depression Scale. *Malaysian Journal of Psychiatry*, **10**, 44–49.

Santos IS, Matijasevich A, Tavares BF, *et al* (2007*a*) Comparing validity of Edinburgh scale and SRQ20 in screening for post-partum depression. *Clinical Practice and Epidemiology in Mental Health*, **3**, 18.

Santos IS, Matijasevich A, Tavares BF, *et al* (2007*b*) Validation of the Edinburgh Postnatal Depression Scale EPDS in a sample of mothers from the 2004 Pelotas Birth Cohort Study. *Cadernos de Saúde Pública*, **23**, 2577–2588.

Schaper AM, Rooney BL, Kay NR, *et al* (1994) Use of the Edinburgh Postnatal Depression Scale to identify postpartum depression in a clinical setting. *Journal of Reproductive Medicine*, **39**, 620–624.

Scottish Intercollegiate Guidelines Network (2002) *SIGN 60: Postnatal Depression and Puerperal Psychosis*. SIGN.

Scottish Intercollegiate Guidelines Network (2012) *SIGN 127: Management of Perinatal Mood Disorders: A National Clinical Guideline*. SIGN.

Seeley S, Murray L, Cooper PJ (1996) Postnatal depression: the outcome for mothers and babies of health visitor intervention. *Health Visitor*, **69**, 135–138.

Seeley S (2001) Postnatal depression and maternal mental health: a public health priority. In *Community Practitioner's & Health Visitors' Association Conference Proceedings, October 2001*, pp. 16–19. CPHVA.

Segre L, Stasik SM, O'Hara MW, *et al* (2010) Listening visits: an evaluation of the effectiveness and acceptability of a home-based depression treatment. *Psychotherapy Research*, **20**, 712–721.

Shafiei T, Small R, McLachlan H (2011) Maternal emotional well-being and the use of health services after childbirth: a study of immigrant women from Afghanistan. *Abstracts from the 4th World Congress on Women's Mental Health, Archives of Women's Mental Health*, **14** (2 suppl), 89–163.

Shakespeare J (2002) Health visitor screening for PND using the EPDS: a process study. *Community Practitioner*, **5**, 381–384.

Shakespeare J, Blake F, Garcia J (2003) A qualitative study of the acceptability of routine screening of postnatal women using the Edinburgh Postnatal Depression Scale. *British Journal of General Practice*, **53**, 614–619.

Sharp D, Hay DF, Pawlby S, *et al* (1995) The impact of postnatal development on boys' intellectual development. *Journal of Child Psychology and Psychiatry*, **36**, 1315–1336.

Sharp DJ, Chew-Graham C, Tylee A, *et al* (2010) A pragmatic randomised controlled trial to compare antidepressants with a community-based psychosocial intervention for the treatment of women with postnatal depression: the RESPOND trial. *Health Technology Assessment*, **14**, 43.

Shereshefsky PM, Lockman RF (1973) Comparison of counselled and non-counselled groups. In *Psychological Aspects of a First Pregnancy and Early Postnatal Adaptation* (eds PM Shereshefsky, LJ Yarrow), pp. 151–163. Raven Press.

Sinclair D, Murray L (1998) Effects of postnatal depression on children's adjustment to school. Teacher's reports. *British Journal of Psychiatry*, **172**, 58–63.

Small R, Johnston V, Orr A (1997) Depression after childbirth: the views of medical students and women compared. *Birth*, **24**, 109–115.

Small R, Lumley J, Yelland J (2003) How useful is the concept of somatisation in cross-cultural studies of maternal depression? A contribution from the Mothers in a New Country (MINC) study. *Journal of Psychosomatic Obstetrics and Gynecology*, **24**, 45–52.

Snaith RP (1983) Pregnancy-related psychiatric disorder. *British Journal of Hospital Medicine*, **29**, 450–456.

Spek V, Nikliček I, Cuijpers P, *et al* (2008) Internet administration of the Edinburgh Depression Scale. *Journal of Affective Disorders*, **106**, 301–305.

Spinelli MG (2003) *Infanticide: Psychosocial and Legal Aspects on Mothers Who Kill*. American Psychiatric Publishing.

Spinelli M, Endicott J (2003) Controlled clinical trial of interpersonal psychotherapy versus parenting education program for depressed pregnant women. *American Journal of Psychiatry*, **160**, 555–562.

Spitzer RL, Endicott J, Robins E (1978) Research Diagnostic Criteria Instrument no. 58. *Archives of General Psychiatry*, **35**, 273–282.

Stamp GE, Crowther CA (1994) Postnatal depression: a South Australian prospective study. *Australian and New Zealand Journal of Obstetrics and Gynaecology*, **34**, 164–167.

Stamp GE, Williams AS, Crowther CA (1995) Evaluation of antenatal and postnatal support to overcome postnatal depression: a randomized, controlled trial. *Birth*, **22**, 138–143.

Steinberg SI, Bellavance F (1999) Characteristics and treatment of women with antenatal and postpartum depression. *International Journal of Psychiatry in Medicine*, **29**, 209–233.

Stern G, Kruckman I (1983) Multi-disciplinary perspectives on postpartum depression: an anthropological critique. *Social Science and Medicine*, **17**, 1027–1041.

Stewart R (2007) Maternal depression and infant growth – a review of recent evidence. *Maternal and Child Nutrition*, **3**, 94–107.

Stewart RC, Umar E, Tomenson B, *et al* (2013) Screening for antenatal depression in Malawi – a comparison of the Edinburgh Postnatal Depression Scale and Self Reporting Questionnaire. *Journal of Affective Disorders*, Jun 13, doi.org/10.106/j.jad.2013.05/036. [Epub ahead of print]

Stuart S, Couser G, Schilder K, *et al* (1998) Post-partum anxiety and depression: onset and comorbidity in a community sample. *Journal of Nervous and Mental Disease*, **186**, 420–424.

Su K-P, Chiu T-H, Huang C-L, *et al* (2007) Different cutoff points for different trimesters? The use of Edinburgh Postnatal Depression Scale and Beck Depression Inventory to screen for depression in pregnant Taiwanese women. *General Hospital Psychiatry*, **29**, 436–441.

Suzuki H (2001) Evolution of the perinatal care system. *Pediatrics International*, **43**, 194–196.

Swalm D, Brooks J, Doherty D, *et al* (2010) Using the Edinburgh Postnatal Depression Scale to screen for anxiety. *Archives of Women's Mental Health*, **13**, 515–522.

Tamaki R, Murata M, Okano T (1997) Risk factors for postpartum depression in Japan. *Psychiatry and Clinical Neuroscience*, **51**, 93–98.

Tandon SD, Cluxton-Keller F, Leis J, *et al* (2012) A comparison of three screening tools to identify perinatal depression among low-income African American women. *Journal of Affective Disorders*, **136**, 155–162.

Taylor E (1989) Postnatal depression: what can a health visitor do? *Journal of Advanced Nursing*, **14**, 877–886.

Taylor S (1998) Instinct or knowledge? *Community Practitioner*, **71**, 427.

Tcixeira JMA, Fisk NM, Glover V (1999) Association between maternal anxiety in pregnancy and increased uterine artery resistance index: cohort based study. *BMJ*, **318**, 153–157.

Teng H-W, Hsu C-S, Shih SM, *et al* (2005) Screening postpartum depression with the Taiwanese version of the Edinburgh Postnatal Depression Scale. *Comprehensive Psychiatry*, **46**, 261–265.

Tesfaye M, Hanlon C, Wondimagegn D, *et al* (2010) Detecting postnatal common mental disorders in Addis Ababa, Ethiopia: validation of the Edinburgh Postnatal Depression Scale and Kessler Scales. *Journal of Affective Disorders*, **122**, 102–108.

Thome M (1991) Emotional distress during the postpartum period from the second to the sixth month, assessed by community nurses. *Nordic Midwifery Research*, **9**, 25–27.

Thome M (1992) Mat heilsugæsluhjúkrunarfræðinga á vanlíðan íslenskra kvenna 2–6 mánuðum eftir barnsburð. [Health nurses assessing distressed Icelandic women 2–6 months postpartum.] *Hjúkrun*, **68**, 8–15.

Thome M (1996) *Distress in Mothers with Difficult Infants in the Community: An Intervention Study*. Doctoral dissertation, Queen Mary College (Edinburgh) and Open University.

Thome M (1999) *Geðheilsuvernd Mæðra Eftir Fæðingu. Greining á vanlíðan með Edinborgarþunglyndiskvarðanum og viðtölum.* [*Mental Protection in Mothers after Childbirth: Analysis of Feeling with the Edinburgh Depression Scale and Interview.*] Rannsóknarstofnun í hjúkrunarfræði og Háskólaútgáfan.

Thome M, Alder B (1999) A telephone intervention to reduce fatigue and symptom distress in mothers with difficult infants in the community. *Journal of Advanced Nursing*, **29**, 128–137.

Thompson WM, Harris B, Lazarus J, *et al* (1998) A comparison of the performance of rating scales used in the diagnosis of postnatal depression. *Acta Psychiatrica Scandinavica*, **98**, 224–227.

Thorpe K, Dragonas T, Golding J (1992) The effects of psychological factors on the mother's emotional well-being during early parenthood: a cross-cultural study of Britain and Greece. *Journal of Reproductive and Infant Psychology*, **10**, 191–248.

Thorpe K (1993) A study of the use of the Edinburgh Postnatal Depression Scale with parent groups outside the postpartum period. *Journal of Reproductive and Infant Psychology*, **11**, 119–125.

Töreki A, Andó B, Keresztúri A, *et al* (2013) The Edinburgh Postnatal Depression Scale: translation and antepartum validation for a Hungarian sample. *Midwifery*, **29**, 308–315.

Tran TD, Tran T, La B, *et al* (2011) Screening for perinatal common mental disorders in women in the north of Vietnam: a comparison of three psychometric instruments. *Journal of Affective Disorders*, **133**, 281–293.

Tran TD, Tran T, Fisher J (2012) Validation of three psychometric instruments for screening for perinatal common mental disorders in men in the north of Vietnam. *Journal of Affective Disorders*, **136**, 104–109.

Uwakwe R, Okonkwo JE (2003) Affective (depressive) morbidity in puerperal Nigerian women: validation of the Edinburgh Postnatal Depression Scale. *Acta Psychiatrica Scandinavica*, **107**, 251–259.

Vega-Dienstmaier JM, Suarez GM, Sanchez MC (2002) Validation of a Spanish version of the Edinburgh Postnatal Depression Scale. *Actas Espanolas de Psiquiatria*, **30**, 106–111.

Vivilaki VG, Dafermos V, Kogevinas M, *et al* (2009) The Edinburgh Postnatal Depression Scale: translation and validation for a Greek sample. *BMC Public Health*, **9**, 329.

Wallis A, Fernandez R, Oprescu F, *et al* (2012) Validation of a Romanian scale to detect antenatal depression. *Central European Journal of Medicine*, **7**, 216–223.

Wang Y, Guo X, Ying L, *et al* (2009) Psychometric evaluation of the Mainland Chinese version of the Edinburgh Postnatal Depression Scale. *International Journal of Nursing Studies*, **46**, 813–823.

Warner R, Appleby L, Whitton A, *et al* (1997) Attitudes toward motherhood in postnatal depression: development of the Maternal Attitudes Questionnaire. *Journal of Psychosomatic Research*, **43**, 351–358.

Watanabe M, Wada K, Sakata Y, *et al* (2008) Maternity blues as predictor of postpartum depression: a prospective cohort study among Japanese women. *Journal of Psychosomatic Obstetrics and Gynaecology*, **29**, 206–212.

Watson JP, Elliott SA, Rugg AJ, *et al* (1984) Psychiatric disorder in pregnancy and the first postnatal year. *British Journal of Psychiatry*, **144**, 453–462.

Webster ML, Thompson JM, Mitchell EA, *et al* (1994) Postnatal depression in a community cohort. *Australian and New Zealand Journal of Psychiatry*, **28**, 42–49.

Webster ML, Linnane JW, Dibley LM, *et al* (2000) Improving antenatal recognition of women at risk for postnatal depression. *Australian and New Zealand Journal of Obstetrics and Gynaecology*, **40**, 409–412.

Wee KY, Skouteris H, Pier C, *et al* (2011) Correlates of ante- and postnatal depression in fathers: a systematic review. *Journal of Affective Disorders*, **130**, 358–377.

Welburn V (1980) *Postnatal Depression*. Collins.

Weobong B, Akpalu B, Doku V, *et al* (2009) The comparative validity of screening scales for postnatal common mental disorder in Kintampo, Ghana. *Journal of Affective Disorders*, **113**, 109–117.

Werrett J, Clifford C (2006) Validation of the Punjabi version of the Edinburgh postnatal depression scale (EPDS). *International Journal of Nursing Studies*, **43**, 227–237.

Whooley MA, Avins AL, Miranda J, *et al* (1997) Case-finding instruments for depression. Two questions are as good as many. *Journal of General Internal Medicine*, **12**, 439–445.

Wickberg B, Hwang CP (1996*a*) The Edinburgh Postnatal Depression Scale: validation on a Swedish community sample. *Acta Psychiatrica Scandinavica*, **94**, 181–184.

Wickberg B, Hwang CP (1996*b*) Counselling of postnatal depression: a controlled study on a population-based Swedish sample. *Journal of Affective Disorders*, **39**, 209–216.

Wickberg B, Hwang CP (1997) Screening for postnatal depression in a population-based Swedish sample. *Acta Psychiatrica Scandinavica*, **95**, 62–66.

Wieck A, Kumar R, Hirst AD, *et al* (1991) Increased sensitivity of dopamine receptors and recurrence of affective psychosis after childbirth. *BMJ*, **303**, 613–616.

Williams C, Cantwell R, Robertson K (2009) *Overcoming Postnatal Depression: A Five Areas Approach*. Hodder & Stoughton.

Williams P, Tarnopolsky A, Hand D (1980) Case definition and case identification in psychiatric epidemiology. *Psychological Medicine*, **10**, 101–114.

Wisner KL, Sit DK, McShea MC, *et al* (2013) Onset timing, thoughts of self-harm, and diagnoses in postpartum women with screen-positive depression findings. *JAMA Psychiatry*, **70**, 490–498.

World Health Organization (1992) *The ICD-10 Classification of Mental and Behavioural Disorders*. WHO.

World Health Organization (1999) *The World Health Report 1999: Making a Difference*. WHO.

Yawn BP, Pace W, Wollan PC, *et al* (2009) Concordance of Edinburgh Postnatal Depression Scale (EPDS) and Patient Health Questionnaire (PHQ-9) to assess increased risk of depression among postpartum women. *Journal of the American Board of Family Medicine*, **22**, 483–491.

Yoshida K, Yamashita H, Ueda M, *et al* (2001) Postnatal depression in Japanese mothers and the reconsideration of 'Satogaeri bunben'. *Pediatrics International*, **43**, 189–193.

Zelkowitz P, Milet TH (1995) Screening for postpartum depression in a community sample. *Canadian Journal of Psychiatry*, **40**, 80–86.

Zigmond AS, Snaith RP (1983) The Hospital Anxiety and Depression Scale. *Acta Psychiatrica Scandinavica*, **67**, 361–370.

Zlotnick C, Johnson SL, Miller IW, *et al* (2001) Postpartum depression in women receiving public assistance: pilot study of an interpersonal-therapy-oriented group intervention. *American Journal of Psychiatry*, **158**, 638–640.

Zung WWK (1965) A self-rating depression scale. *Archives of General Psychiatry*, **12**, 63–70.

Index

Compiled by Linda English